Renal Diet

Cookbook

for Beginners

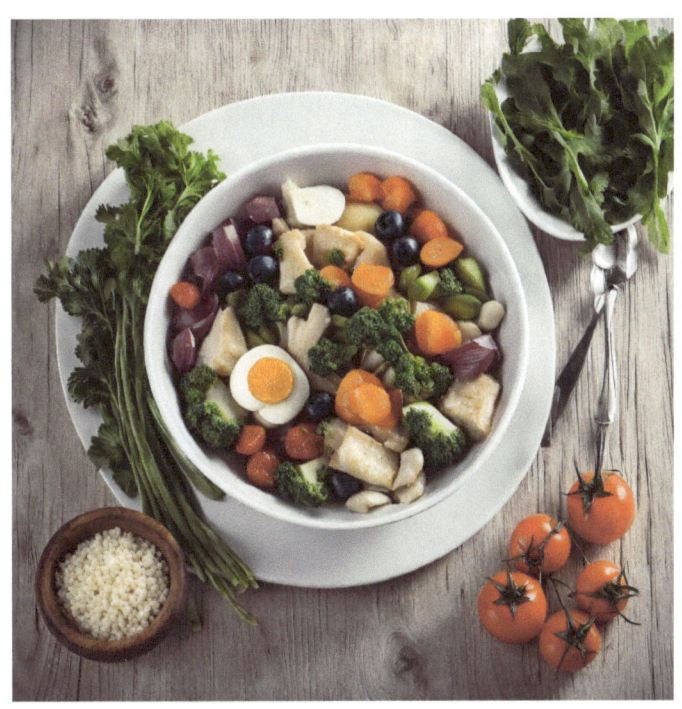

Delicious Low sodium recipes for kidney Diseases prevention and sound kidney health

Michael S. White

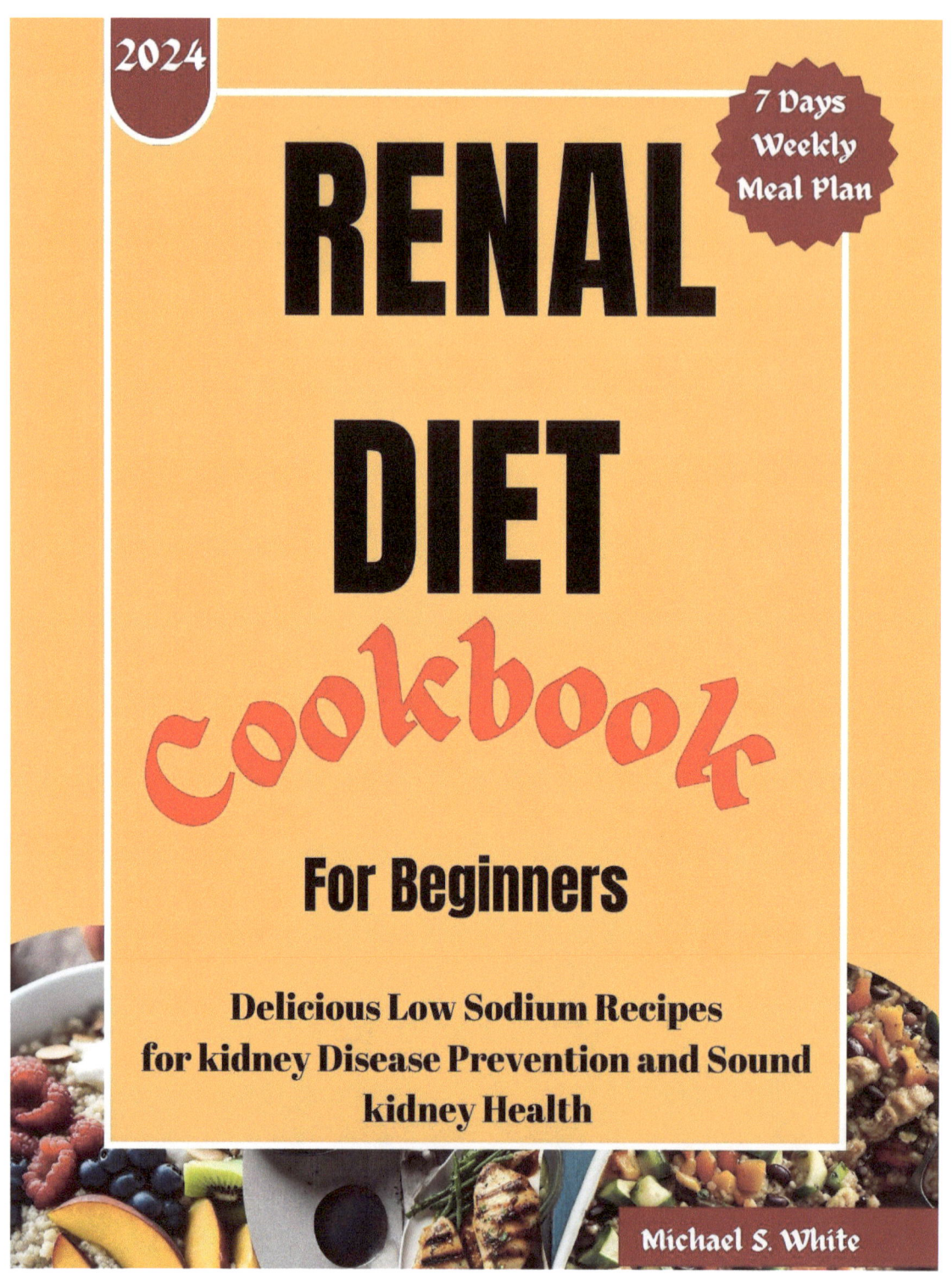

2024

RENAL

DIET

Cookbook

For Beginners

7 Days Weekly Meal Plan

**Delicious Low Sodium Recipes
for kidney Disease Prevention and Sound
kidney Health**

Michael S. White

Copyright © 2024 by Michael S White

Table of Content

Chapter 7: Beverages to Quench and Protect

Hydrating and Kidney-Supportive Drinks

Low Sodium Infusions and Smoothies

    1. Citrus Mint Infused Water:

    2. Berry Blast Smoothie:

Herbal Teas for Kidney Wellness

    1. Hibiscus Rosehip Tea:

    2. Nettle Leaf Infusion:

Chapter 8: Meal Plans and Weekly Menus

Sample Meal Plans for a Week

Day 1

    Breakfast - Oatmeal with Berries and Almonds:

    Lunch - Chicken and Vegetable Stir-Fry:

    Dinner - Baked Salmon with Quinoa and Asparagus:

Day 2

    Breakfast - Spinach and Feta Omelette:

    Lunch - Lentil Soup with Vegetables:

    Dinner - Grilled Chicken with Sweet Potato Mash:

Day 3

    Breakfast - Greek Yogurt Parfait:

    Lunch - Quinoa and Black Bean Salad:

    Dinner - Turkey and Vegetable Skewers with Brown Rice:

Day 4

Breakfast - Veggie Omelette with Whole Grain Toast

    Lunch - Chickpea Salad with Cucumber and Avocado:

    Dinner - Shrimp Stir-Fry with Broccoli and Brown Rice:

Day 5

    Breakfast - Blueberry Banana Smoothie Bowl:

    Lunch - Spinach and Lentil Salad with Balsamic Vinaigrette:

    Dinner - Grilled Vegetable and Chicken Skewers with Quinoa:

Day 6:

    Breakfast - Chia Seed Pudding with Fresh Fruit:

    Lunch - Turkey and Avocado Wrap:

    Dinner - Baked Cod with Lemon and Herbs, Quinoa, and Steamed Broccoli:

Day 7

    Breakfast - Overnight Oats with Nut Butter and Banana:

    Lunch - Quinoa Stuffed Bell Peppers:

    Dinner - Eggplant and Chickpea Curry with Brown Rice:

Preface

Greetings and welcome to the educational "Renal Disease Prevention Cookbook." My goal as the author is to lead you through a story that combines the ease of tasty, nourishing dishes with the complexity of kidney health. This cookbook is a guide to knowing, appreciating, and actively supporting kidney health—it's more than just a compilation of recipes.

Introduction

Understanding Kidney Health

Kidney health is a cornerstone of overall well-being, playing a pivotal role in maintaining balance within the body. These bean-shaped organs, nestled beneath the rib cage, are not only responsible for filtering waste and excess fluids from the blood but also play crucial roles in blood pressure regulation, electrolyte balance, and red blood cell production.

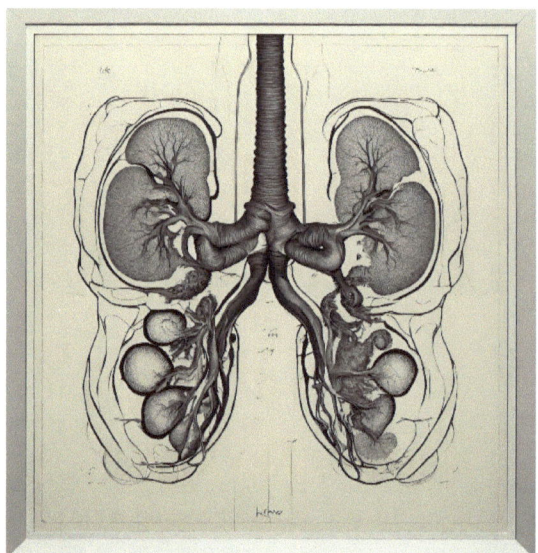

Anatomy and Function:

The kidneys, comprising millions of tiny structures called nephrons, filter blood to remove waste, toxins, and extra fluids. This intricate system ensures that essential substances, such as electrolytes and proteins, are retained while waste is directed to the bladder as urine. Beyond filtration, kidneys also release hormones like erythropoietin to stimulate red blood cell production and renin to regulate blood pressure.

Blood Pressure Regulation:

The intricate relationship between kidneys and blood pressure involves the renin-angiotensin-aldosterone system. When blood pressure drops, the kidneys release renin, initiating a cascade that ultimately leads to the retention of sodium and water, raising blood pressure. Conversely, if blood pressure is elevated, the kidneys adjust to excrete excess sodium and fluids, helping to lower pressure.

Electrolyte Balance:

Kidneys maintain a delicate balance of electrolytes like sodium, potassium, and calcium. This equilibrium is crucial for nerve function, muscle contractions, and overall cellular health. Any disruption in these levels can lead to complications affecting the heart, muscles, and nervous system.

Common Kidney Disorders:

Understanding kidney health involves awareness of common disorders, such as chronic kidney disease (CKD), kidney stones, and infections. CKD, often a progressive condition, can result from various factors, including diabetes and hypertension. Kidney stones, formed from mineral and acid deposits, can cause intense pain when passing through the urinary tract.

Lifestyle Factors for Kidney Health:

Maintaining kidney health extends beyond medical considerations. Adopting a healthy lifestyle significantly contributes to their well-being. Staying hydrated, consuming a balanced diet rich in fruits, vegetables, and whole grains, managing blood pressure, and avoiding excessive salt intake are fundamental practices.

Regular Monitoring and Seeking Medical Advice:

Routine check-ups that include blood pressure measurement and kidney function tests are essential for early detection of any issues. Individuals with risk factors such as diabetes or a family history of kidney disease should be particularly vigilant. Seeking prompt medical advice when symptoms like changes in urine color, swelling, or persistent fatigue occur is crucial for timely intervention.

Understanding kidney health is empowering; it enables individuals to make informed choices that positively impact their overall well-being. From the intricacies of nephron function to the significance of lifestyle choices, this understanding forms the foundation for a proactive approach to kidney health, fostering a life of vitality and longevity.

Importance of Low Sodium Diets

A diet reduced in salt is very important for general health, especially when it comes to managing and preventing many types of illnesses. Although excessive sodium intake, as is frequently seen in modern diets, can have negative effects, sodium is an important electrolyte for body processes. An examination of the significance of switching to a low-sodium diet is provided below:

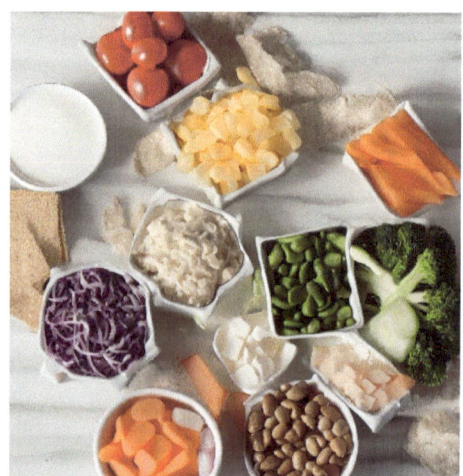

Control of Blood Pressure:
Elevated blood pressure is directly correlated with high sodium intake. A diet high in sodium can cause fluid retention, which raises blood pressure by filling the vessels with more blood. Hypertension, or persistently high blood pressure, is a major risk factor for renal disease, heart disease, and stroke.

Renal Health:

The body's salt equilibrium is critically dependent on the kidneys. A diet heavy in salt can potentially strain the kidneys. eventually resulting in diminished function. A low-sodium diet is frequently advised for people with renal diseases or those who are at risk of developing kidney difficulties in order to lessen the strain on these organs.

Flowing Equilibrium:

Sodium and the body's fluid equilibrium are closely related. This equilibrium can be upset by high sodium levels, which can lead to fluid retention. Edema, often known as edema, is a typical side effect of consuming too much sodium. It can affect any area of the body, although it usually affects the hands, ankles, and legs.

Heart Health:

Beyond controlling blood pressure, heart health can be greatly enhanced by eating a low-sodium diet. Consuming too much sodium raises the risk of heart disease, heart attacks, and strokes by hardening and narrowing the arteries.

Joint Health:

Excessive sodium intake may contribute to inflammation and exacerbate conditions like arthritis. By adopting a low sodium diet, individuals may experience reduced joint pain and inflammation.

Improved Overall Well-being:

Beyond specific health conditions, a low sodium diet contributes to overall well-being. It encourages the consumption of nutrient-dense foods, such as fruits, vegetables, and whole grains, fostering a balanced and heart-healthy approach to nutrition.

In essence, a low sodium diet is a cornerstone of preventive health measures. It empowers individuals to take control of their cardiovascular and renal health, reduce the risk of chronic diseases, and promote a vibrant and energetic life. Making mindful choices about sodium intake is an investment in long-term well-being and a crucial step towards a healthier and more fulfilling lifestyle.

Chapter 1 : The Foundation of Renal-Friendly Cooking

Renal disease prevention is a critical aspect of overall health, and adopting a renal-friendly cooking approach lays the groundwork for safeguarding kidney function. Let's delve into the foundational principles of renal disease prevention and how they form the cornerstone of a renal-friendly cooking journey.

Understanding Renal Disease:

Renal disease encompasses a spectrum of conditions affecting the kidneys, ranging from acute issues to chronic conditions like chronic kidney disease (CKD). The kidneys, vital for filtering waste and excess fluids, face various challenges that can impair their function. Hypertension, diabetes, and genetic factors are among the contributors to renal issues.

Key Nutritional Considerations:

Renal disease prevention through nutrition involves strategic choices to support kidney health. Key considerations include:

Sodium Restriction: Limiting sodium intake is crucial to manage blood pressure and reduce strain on the kidneys. Renal-friendly cooking prioritizes herbs, spices, and other flavor enhancers over high-sodium additives.

Protein Moderation: Controlling protein intake helps manage the workload on the kidneys. Renal-friendly cooking emphasizes lean protein sources and appropriate portion sizes.
Fluid Balance: Maintaining proper hydration is vital. Renal-friendly cooking incorporates foods with high water content and mindful fluid management.

Phosphorus and Potassium Control: Monitoring phosphorus and potassium levels is essential for individuals with kidney issues. Renal-friendly cooking involves choosing foods that align with these dietary restrictions.

Tips for Creating Kidney-Friendly Meals:

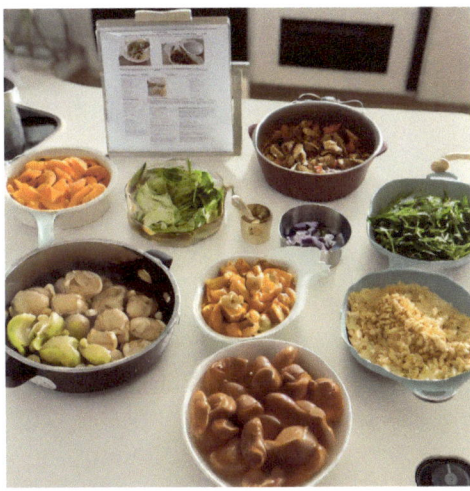

Fresh Ingredients: Prioritize fresh fruits and vegetables, lean proteins, and whole grains. These form the basis of nutritious and kidney-friendly meals.

Herbs and Spices: Elevate flavors without sodium by using a variety of herbs and spices. This not only enhances taste but also contributes to the overall appeal of renal-friendly dishes.

Balanced Plate Approach: Create balanced meals that include a mix of proteins, grains, and colorful vegetables. This ensures a well-rounded nutritional profile.

Mindful Cooking Techniques: Opt for cooking methods that retain nutrients and minimize added fats, such as steaming, baking, and grilling.

Empowering Lifestyle Choices:
Renal disease prevention extends beyond the kitchen to lifestyle choices. Regular exercise, maintaining a healthy weight, and managing conditions like diabetes and hypertension contribute significantly to kidney health.

The foundation of renal-friendly cooking is rooted in the proactive prevention of renal disease. By understanding the nuances of kidney health, making informed nutritional choices, and embracing a holistic approach to well-being, individuals can embark on a culinary journey that not only supports their kidneys but also promotes overall health and vitality. Renal-friendly cooking is a powerful tool in the arsenal of preventive health measures, fostering a lifestyle that prioritizes the longevity and optimal function of these vital organs.

Chapter 2: Breakfast Boosters

Energizing and Nutrient-Packed Morning Recipes

Low Sodium Breakfast Smoothies

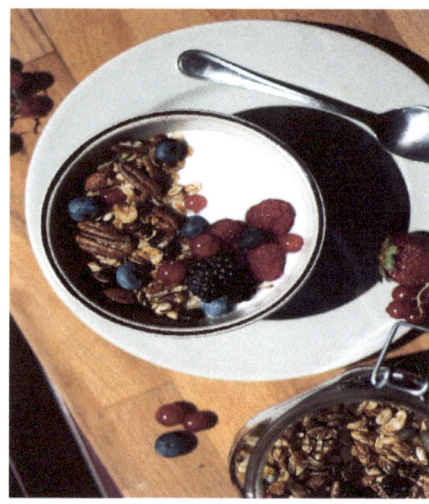

Serving: 2 servings

Duration: 5 minutes

Ingredients:

1 cup fresh berries (strawberries, blueberries, or raspberries)

1 banana, peeled and sliced

1 cup spinach leaves, washed

1/2 cup low-fat yogurt

1 tablespoon chia seeds

1 cup ice cubes

1 cup water or low-sodium fruit juice

Directions:

- In a blender, combine berries, banana, spinach, yogurt, chia seeds, and ice cubes.
- Add water or low-sodium fruit juice to achieve your desired consistency.
- Blend until smooth and creamy.
- Pour into glasses and enjoy this refreshing low sodium breakfast smoothie, packed with antioxidants and kidney-friendly nutrients.

Protein-Packed Breakfast Bowls

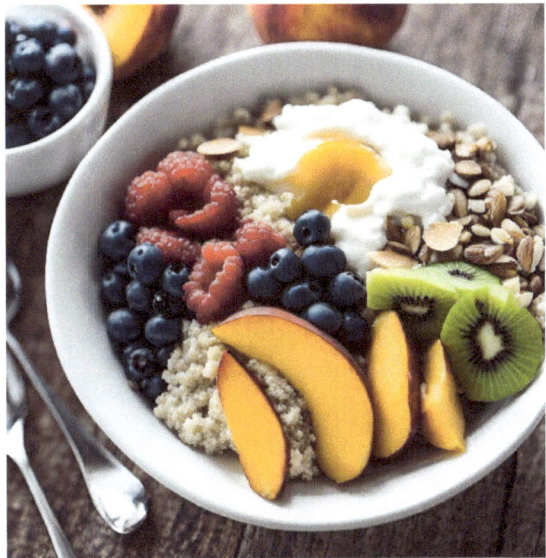

Serving: 2 servings

Duration: 15 minutes

Ingredients:

1 cup quinoa, cooked

1 cup low-fat cottage cheese

1 cup mixed fresh fruit (such as sliced peaches, kiwi, and berries)

1/4 cup almonds, chopped

1 tablespoon honey

1 teaspoon cinnamon

Directions:

- Divide the cooked quinoa between two bowls.
- Top each bowl with half of the cottage cheese.
- Arrange the mixed fresh fruit on top.
- Sprinkle chopped almonds over the fruit.
- Drizzle honey over each bowl and sprinkle with cinnamon.
- Gently mix the ingredients in each bowl just before eating to enjoy a protein-packed and kidney-friendly breakfast.

These energizing and nutrient-packed recipes not only cater to renal health but also bring a burst of flavors to your morning routine. Incorporate them into your breakfast repertoire for a delicious and nourishing start to the day.

Chapter 3: Lunchtime Delights

Satisfying and Nourishing Midday Meals

Welcome to the heart of your day with "Satisfying and Nourishing Midday Meals." This section is dedicated to elevating your lunch experience with vibrant salads featuring renal-friendly dressings and delectable low-sodium wraps and sandwiches.

Salads with Renal-Friendly Dressings

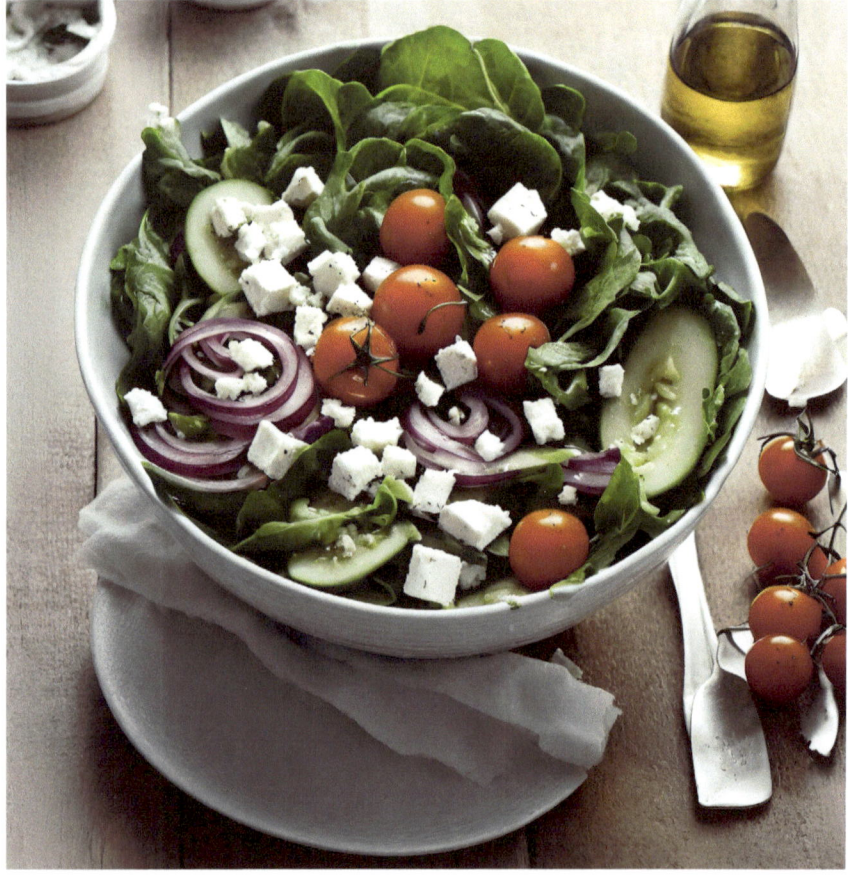

Serving: 2 servings

Duration: 15 minutes

Ingredients:

4 cups mixed salad greens (lettuce, spinach, arugula)

1 cup cherry tomatoes, halved

1/2 cucumber, sliced

1/4 cup red onion, thinly sliced

1/4 cup crumbled feta cheese

2 tablespoons olive oil

1 tablespoon balsamic vinegar

1 teaspoon honey

Salt and pepper to taste

Directions:

- In a large bowl, combine mixed salad greens, cherry tomatoes, cucumber, red onion, and feta cheese.
- In a small bowl, whisk together olive oil, balsamic vinegar, honey, salt, and pepper to create the renal-friendly dressing.
- Drizzle the dressing over the salad and toss gently to coat evenly.
- Divide into two servings, and enjoy a refreshing and nourishing salad that supports kidney health.

Flavorful Low Sodium Wraps and Sandwiches

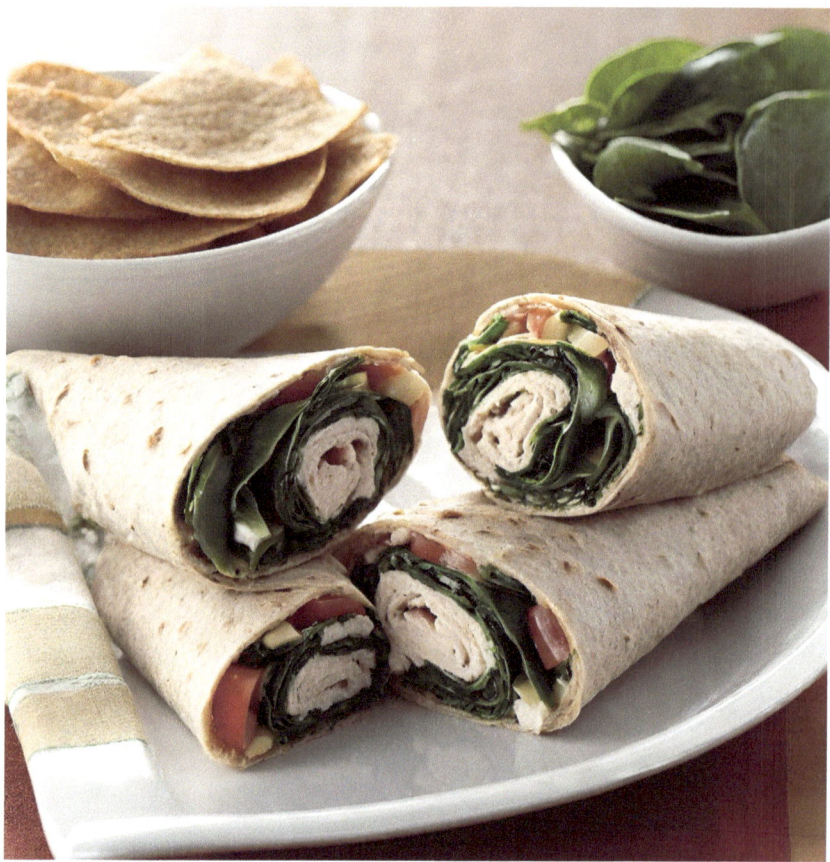

Serving: 2 servings

Duration: 10 minutes

Ingredients:

4 whole-grain wraps or slices of low-sodium bread

1/2 pound deli-sliced turkey or chicken

1 cup fresh spinach leaves

1 medium tomato, thinly sliced

1/4 cup hummus

1 tablespoon Dijon mustard

1/2 avocado, sliced

Directions:

- Lay out the wraps or bread slices.
- Spread hummus on each wrap or bread slice, followed by Dijon mustard.
- Layer the deli-sliced turkey or chicken, fresh spinach leaves, tomato slices, and avocado.

- Roll up the wraps or assemble the sandwiches.
- Slice in half and serve, creating a flavorful and low sodium midday meal that's not only satisfying but also supportive of kidney health.

These midday meals are not just about nourishing your body but also indulging your taste buds. With kidney-friendly ingredients and thoughtful preparation, your lunchtime experience becomes a delightful and health-conscious celebration. Enjoy the goodness with every bite!

Chapter 4: Dinner Classics Reinvented

Wholesome Dinners for Optimal Kidney Health

Dive into the realm of "Wholesome Dinners for Optimal Kidney Health," where we explore the richness of renal-friendly casseroles and one-pot meals, along with the sizzling satisfaction of grilled delights featuring low sodium marinades.

Renal-Friendly Casseroles and One-Pot Meals

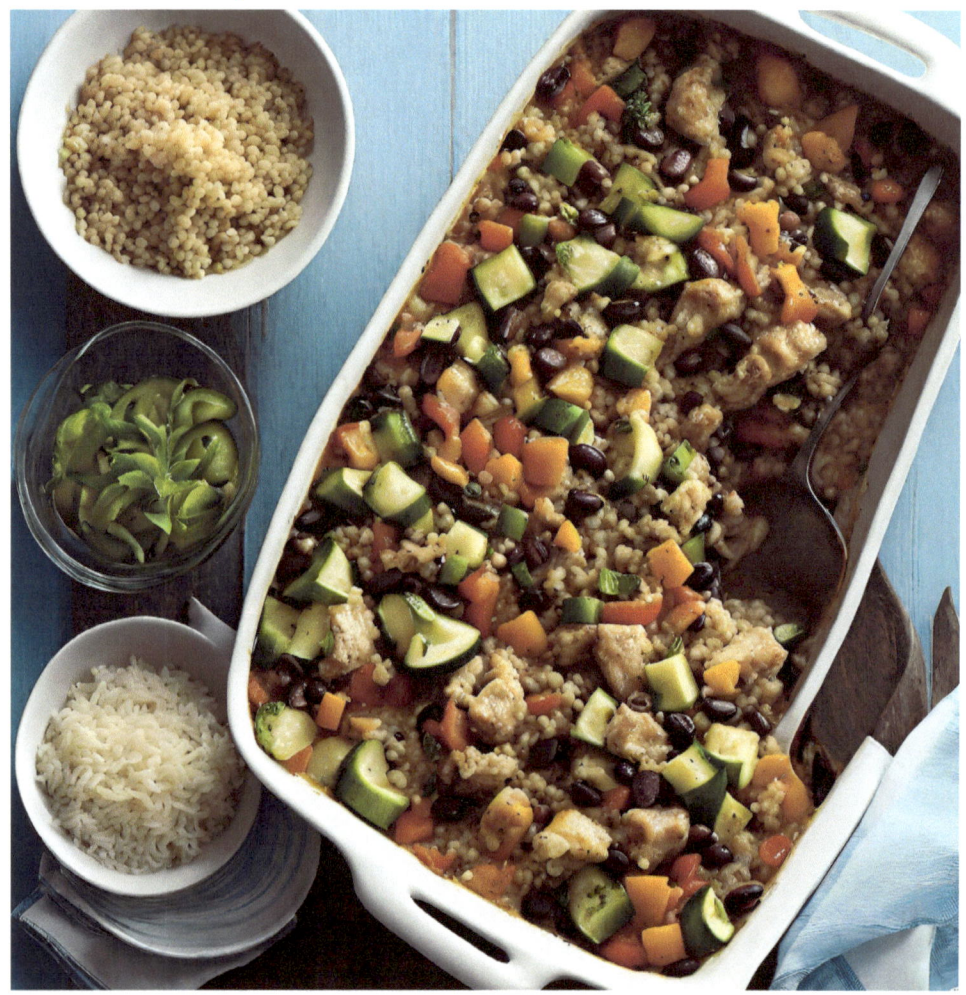

Serving: 4 servings

Duration: 45 minutes

Ingredients:

1 pound lean protein (chicken, turkey, or tofu), diced

2 cups brown rice, cooked

1 can low-sodium black beans, drained and rinsed

1 cup mixed vegetables (bell peppers, zucchini, carrots), diced

1 cup low-sodium chicken or vegetable broth

1 teaspoon garlic powder

1 teaspoon onion powder

1 teaspoon cumin

Salt and pepper to taste

Fresh cilantro for garnish

Directions:

- Preheat the oven to 375°F (190°C).
- In a large bowl, combine diced protein, cooked brown rice, black beans, mixed vegetables, garlic powder, onion powder, cumin, salt, and pepper.
- Transfer the mixture to a casserole dish or a deep skillet.
- Pour low-sodium chicken or vegetable broth over the ingredients.
- Bake for 30-35 minutes or until the protein is cooked through and the vegetables are tender.
- Garnish with fresh cilantro and serve, savoring a wholesome dinner that nurtures kidney health.

Grilled Delights with Low Sodium Marinades

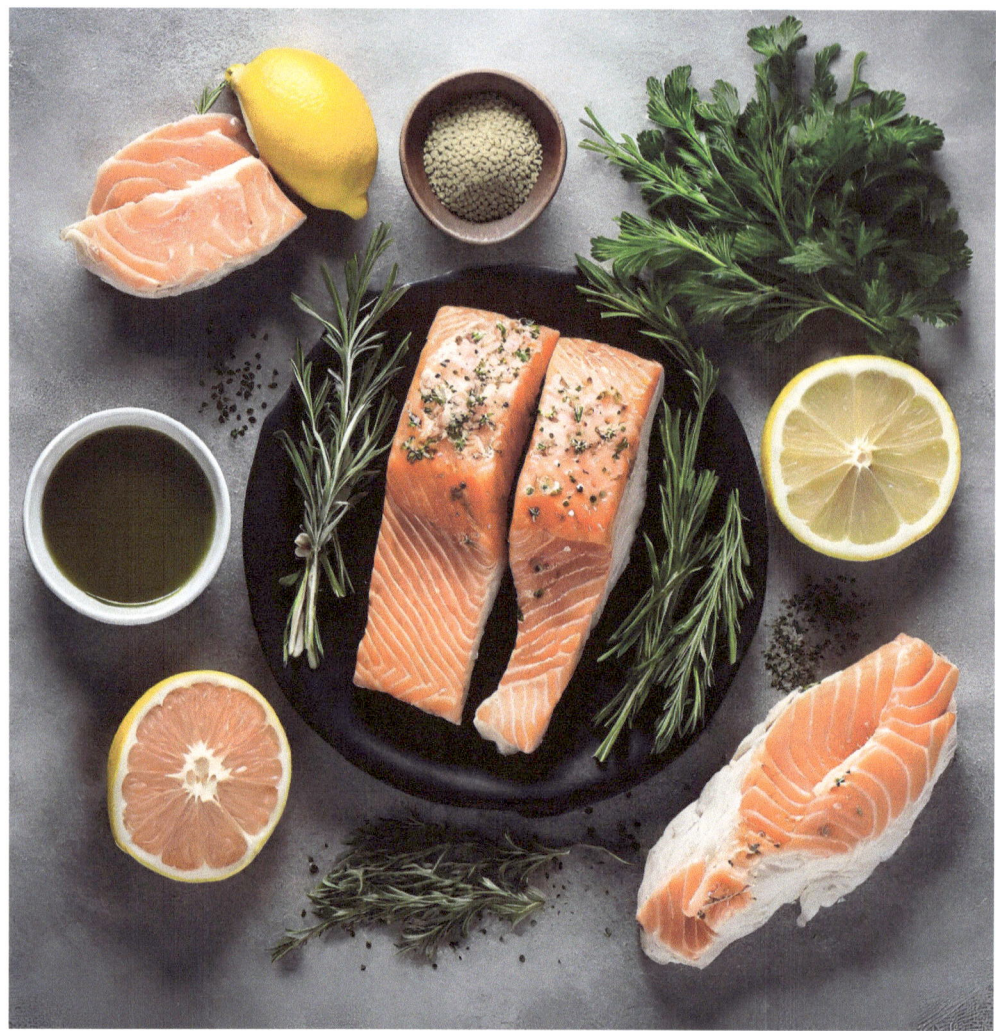

Serving: 4 servings

Duration: 30 minutes

Ingredients:

1 pound lean protein (salmon, chicken, or tofu)

2 tablespoons low-sodium soy sauce

1 tablespoon olive oil

1 tablespoon lemon juice

1 teaspoon garlic powder

1 teaspoon dried herbs (rosemary, thyme, or oregano)

1/2 teaspoon black pepper

Fresh herbs for garnish (parsley or cilantro)

Directions:

- In a bowl, whisk together low-sodium soy sauce, olive oil, lemon juice, garlic powder, dried herbs, and black pepper to create a kidney-friendly marinade.
- Place the protein in a shallow dish and pour the marinade over it.
- Allow the protein to marinate for at least 15 minutes.
- Preheat the grill to medium-high heat.
- Grill the protein for 6-8 minutes per side or until fully cooked.
- Garnish with fresh herbs and serve, relishing in the flavors of grilled delights with a low sodium twist.

These dinner options not only prioritize kidney health but also elevate your dining experience with a variety of flavors and textures. From comforting casseroles to sizzling grilled dishes, each bite is a step towards a balanced and nourished life. Enjoy the journey to optimal kidney health through wholesome and delectable dinners!

Chapter 5: Snack Attack

Kidney–Friendly Snacks for Anytime Cravings

Indulge in guilt-free snacking with "Kidney-Friendly Snacks for Anytime Cravings," offering an array of crunchy and savory options along with sweet treats carefully crafted to satisfy your snack cravings without compromising kidney health.

Crunchy and Savory Options

Serving: 2 servings per recipe

Duration: Varies by recipe

1. Roasted Chickpeas:

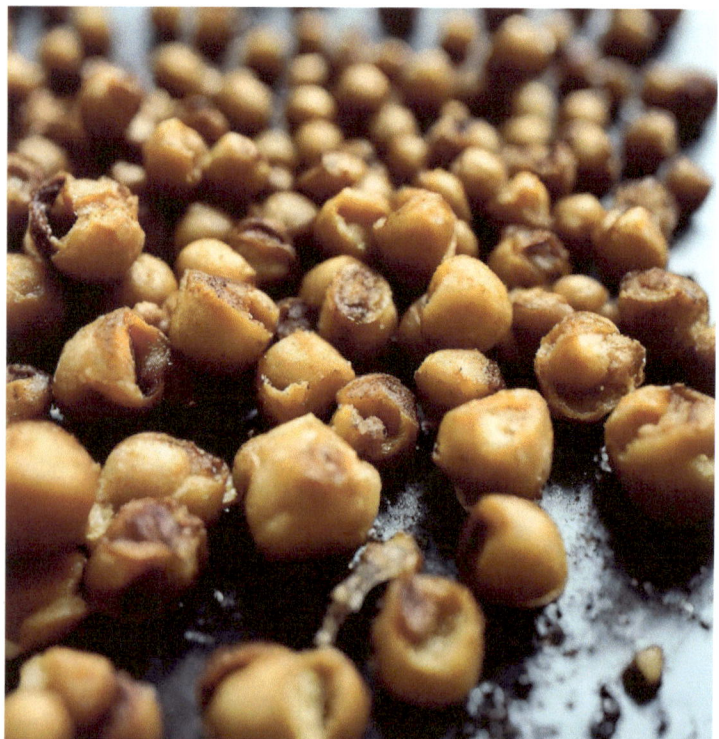

Ingredients:
1 can chickpeas, drained and rinsed
1 tablespoon olive oil
1 teaspoon cumin
1/2 teaspoon paprika
Salt to taste

Directions:

- Preheat the oven to 400°F (200°C).
- In a bowl, toss chickpeas with olive oil, cumin, paprika, and salt.
- Spread chickpeas on a baking sheet and roast for 25-30 minutes until crispy.

2. Veggie Sticks with Hummus:

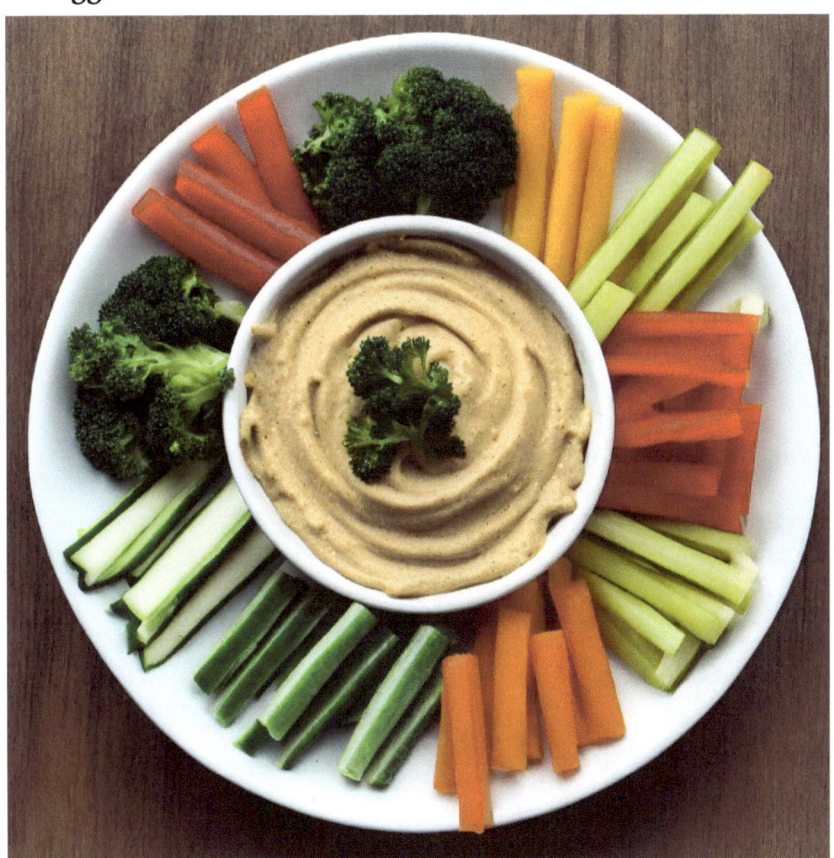

Ingredients:

Carrot sticks, cucumber slices, bell pepper strips
1/2 cup low-sodium hummus

Directions:

- Arrange veggie sticks on a plate.
- Serve with a side of low-sodium hummus for a satisfying and crunchy snack.

Sweet Treats with Reduced Sodium

Serving: 2 servings per recipe

Duration: Varies by recipe

1. Fruit Kabobs:

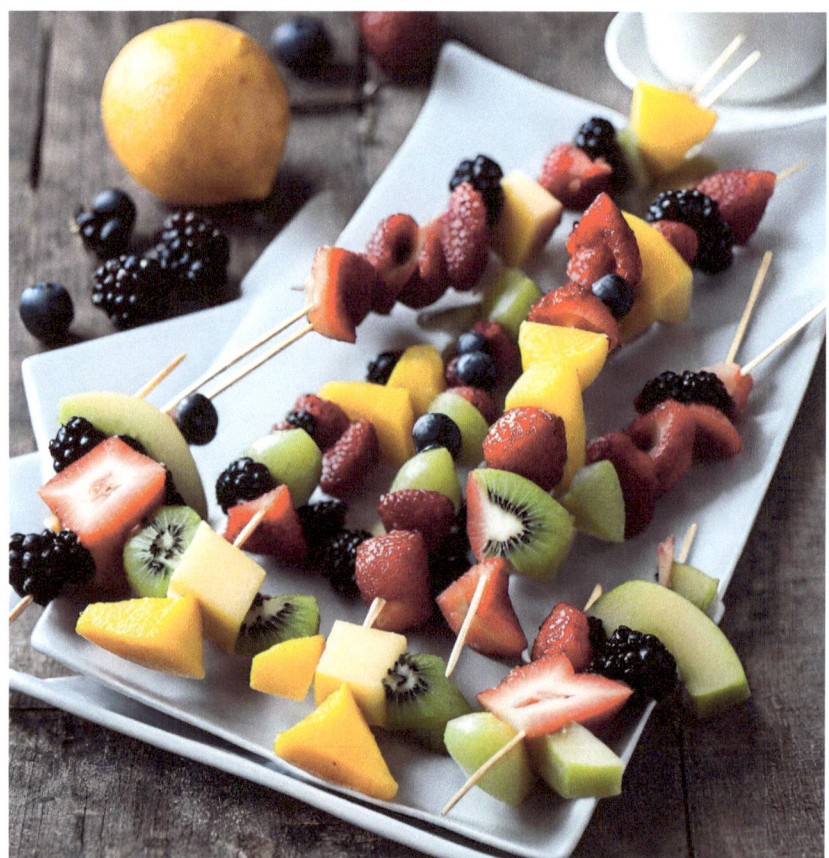

Ingredients:
Fresh fruit chunks (melon, berries, pineapple)
1 tablespoon honey (optional)

Directions:
- Thread fruit chunks onto skewers.
- Drizzle with honey if desired and enjoy a naturally sweet and low sodium treat.

2. Greek Yogurt Parfait:

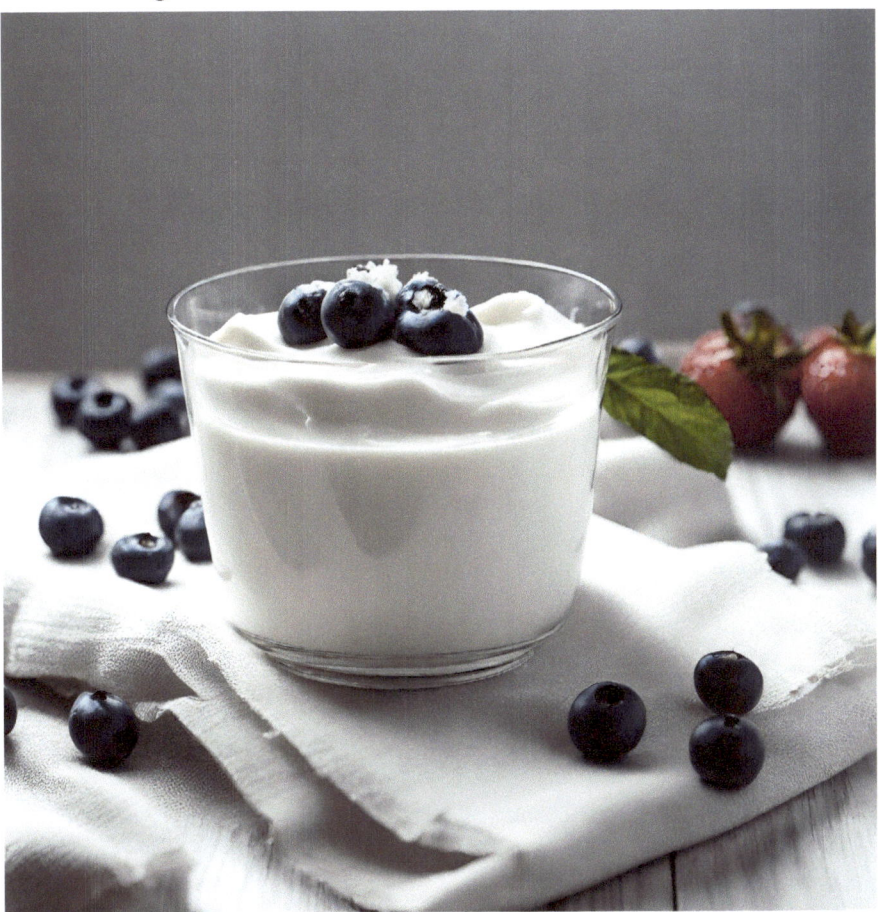

Ingredients:
1 cup low-sodium Greek yogurt
1/2 cup fresh berries
2 tablespoons chopped nuts
1 tablespoon honey (optional)

Directions:
- In a glass, layer Greek yogurt, fresh berries, and chopped nuts.
- Drizzle with honey if desired, creating a delicious and kidney-friendly parfait.

These snacks not only curb your cravings but also contribute to kidney health. Whether you're in the mood for a savory crunch or a sweet delight, these options are tailored to provide satisfaction without compromising your commitment to optimal renal wellness. Enjoy these anytime snacks guilt-free!

Chapter 6: Desserts for Kidney Health

Indulgent yet Healthy Sweets

Satisfy your sweet tooth guilt-free with "Indulgent yet Healthy Sweets," featuring a collection of low sodium dessert recipes and creative fruit-based delights that promise a delightful experience without compromising your commitment to health.

Low Sodium Dessert Recipes

Serving: 4 servings per recipe

Duration: Varies by recipe

1. Chia Seed Pudding:

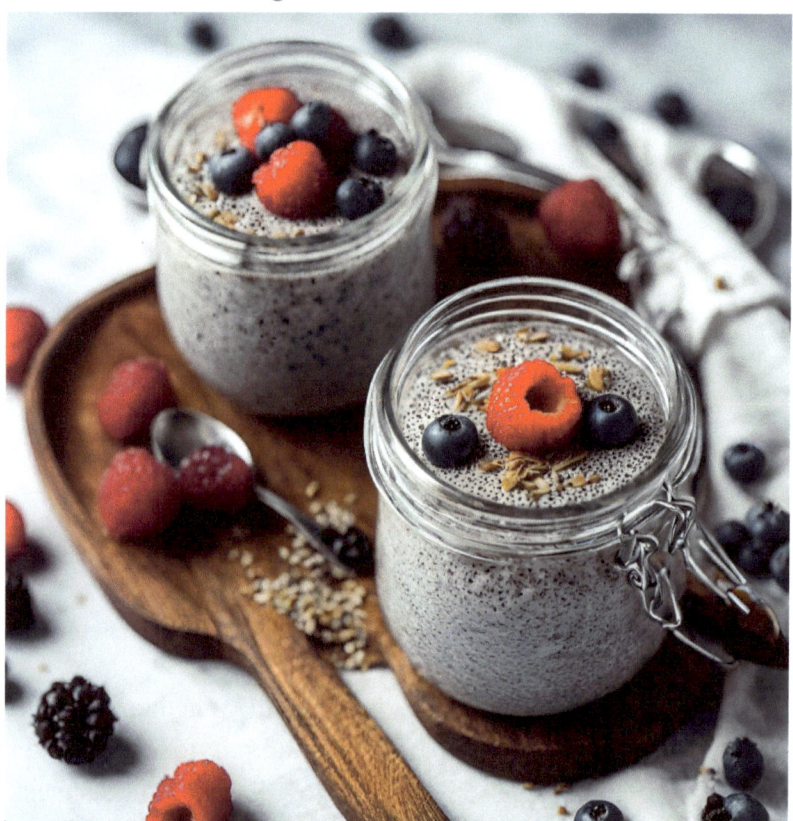

Ingredients:
1/4 cup chia seeds
1 cup low-sodium almond milk
1 tablespoon maple syrup

1/2 teaspoon vanilla extract

Directions:

- In a bowl, mix chia seeds, almond milk, maple syrup, and vanilla extract.
- Refrigerate for at least 4 hours or overnight.
- Serve chilled, garnished with fresh berries or a sprinkle of cinnamon.

2. Baked Apples with Cinnamon:

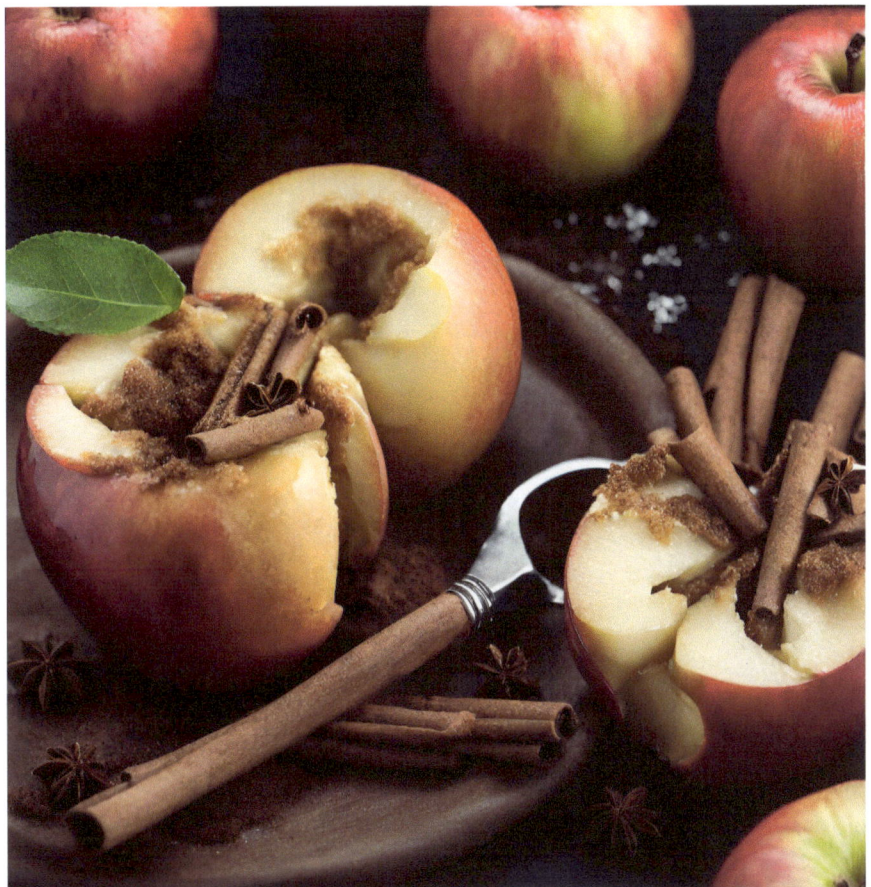

Ingredients:

2 apples, cored and halved

1 teaspoon cinnamon

1 tablespoon chopped nuts (walnuts or almonds)

1 tablespoon honey (optional)

Directions:

- Preheat the oven to 375°F (190°C).
- Place apple halves on a baking sheet.
- Sprinkle it with cinnamon and chopped nuts.

- Bake for 20-25 minutes until the apples are tender.
- Drizzle with honey if desired and serve warm.

Creative Fruit-Based Desserts

Serving: 4 servings per recipe

Duration: Varies by recipe

1. Watermelon Pizza:

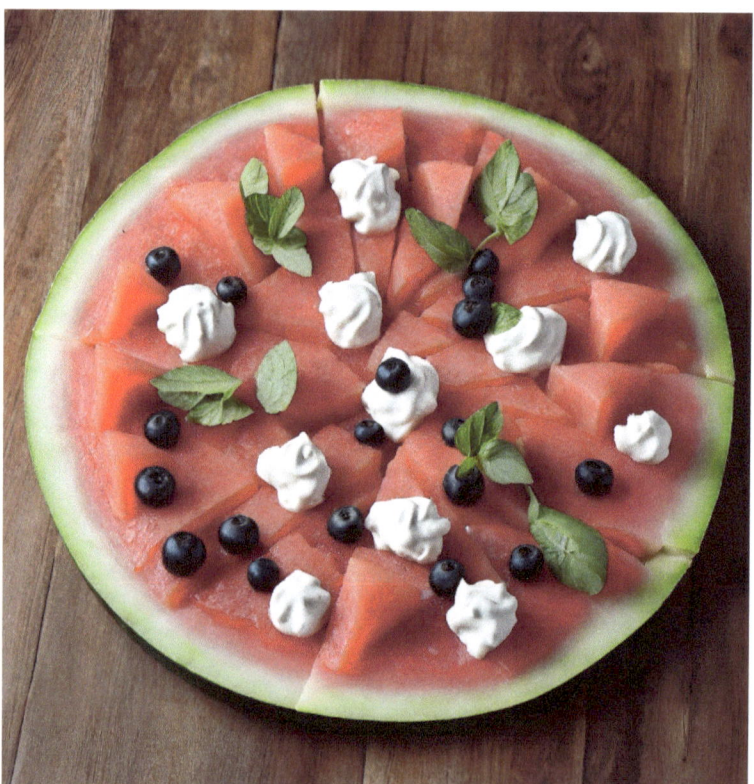

Ingredients:
1 slice of watermelon (1-inch thick)
1/2 cup low-fat Greek yogurt
Assorted fresh fruits (strawberries, kiwi, blueberries)

Directions:
- Cut a slice of watermelon into a pizza shape.
- Spread Greek yogurt over the watermelon slice.
- Top with assorted fresh fruits for a colorful and refreshing fruit pizza.

2. Grilled Pineapple with Mint:

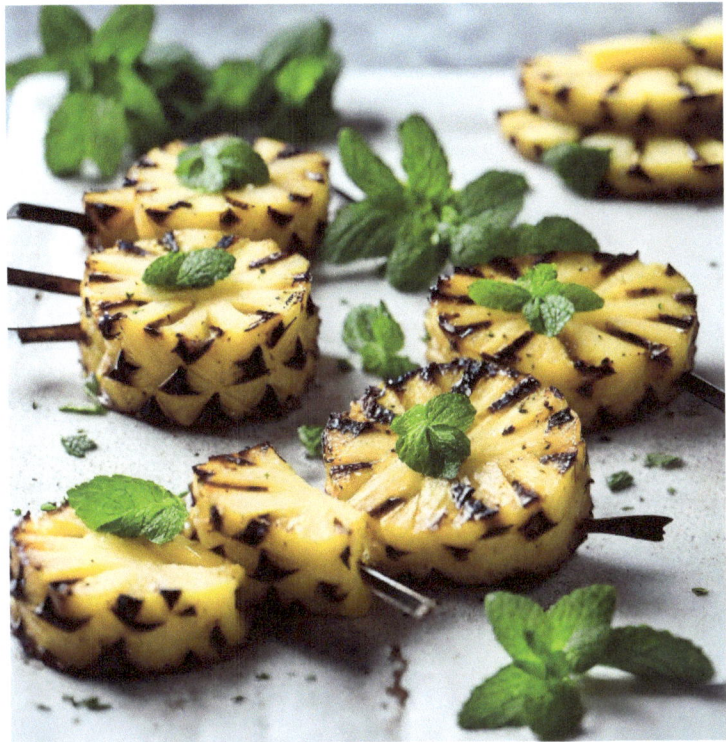

Ingredients:
4 pineapple slices
1 tablespoon fresh mint, chopped
1 teaspoon lime juice

Directions:
- Preheat the grill or grill pan.
- Grill pineapple slices for 2-3 minutes per side.
- Sprinkle with fresh mint and drizzle with lime juice before serving.

These indulgent yet healthy sweets redefine dessert time by combining sweetness with nourishment. Whether you opt for a comforting chia seed pudding or a refreshing watermelon pizza, each recipe promises a delightful and health-conscious treat. Enjoy the indulgence without compromising on your commitment to a balanced and wholesome lifestyle!

Chapter 7: Beverages to Quench and Protect

Hydrating and Kidney-Supportive Drinks

Quench your thirst and support your kidneys with "Hydrating and Kidney-Supportive Drinks," featuring low sodium infusions, refreshing smoothies, and herbal teas specially curated to promote hydration and overall renal wellness.

Low Sodium Infusions and Smoothies

Serving: 2 servings per recipe

Duration: Varies by recipe

1. Citrus Mint Infused Water:

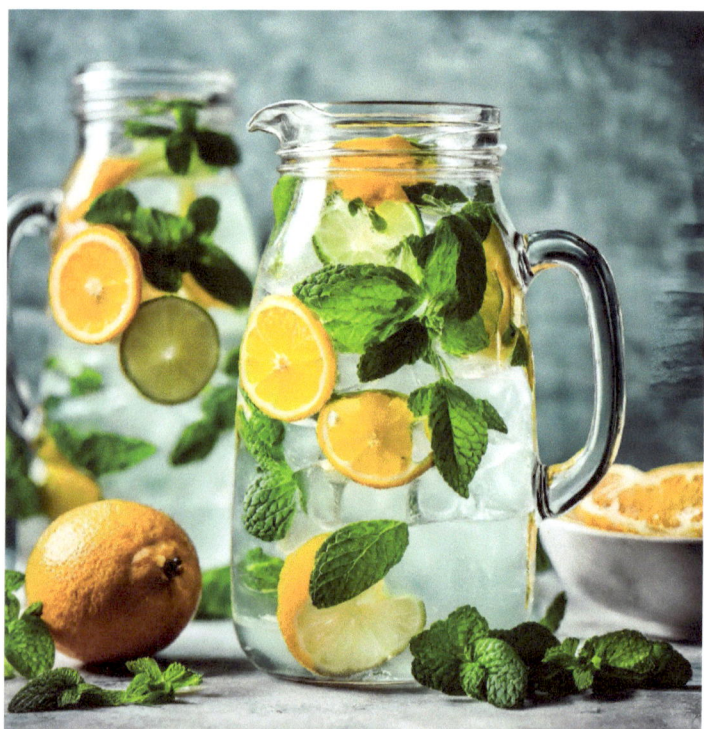

Ingredients:
1 lemon, thinly sliced
1 lime, thinly sliced
1/2 cup fresh mint leaves
1 liter water

Directions:

- Combine lemon slices, lime slices, and mint leaves in a pitcher.
- Fill the pitcher with water and refrigerate for at least 2 hours.
- Serve over ice for a refreshing and low sodium citrus mint infusion.

2. Berry Blast Smoothie:

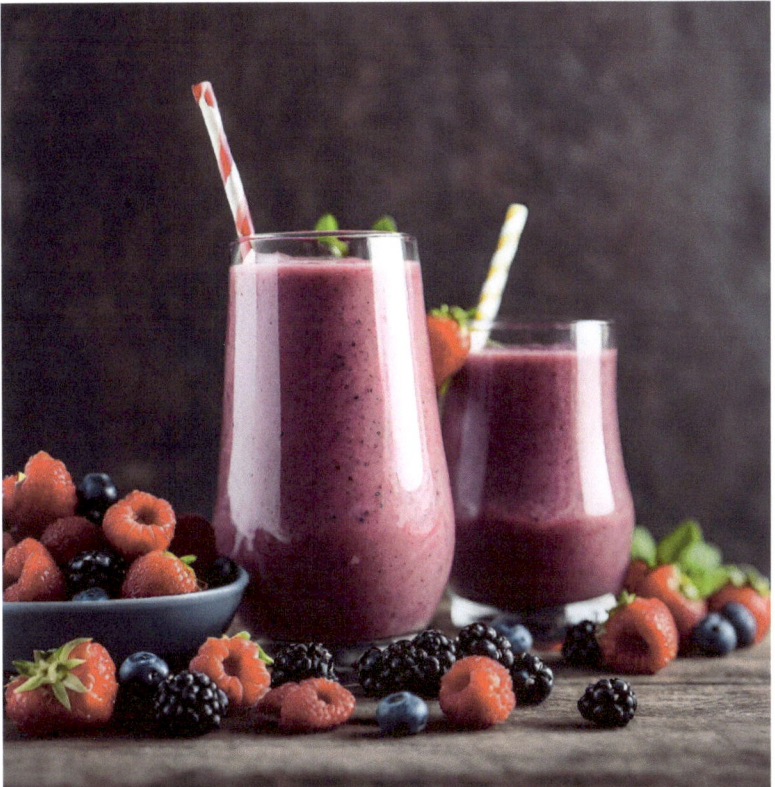

Ingredients:

1 cup mixed berries (strawberries, blueberries, raspberries)

1/2 banana, peeled and sliced

1 cup low-sodium coconut water

1/2 cup low-fat Greek yogurt

1 tablespoon chia seeds

Directions:

- In a blender, combine mixed berries, banana, coconut water, Greek yogurt, and chia seeds.
- Blend until smooth and creamy.
- Pour into glasses and enjoy a hydrating and kidney-supportive berry blast.

Herbal Teas for Kidney Wellness

Serving: 1 cup per recipe

Duration: Varies by recipe

1. Hibiscus Rosehip Tea:

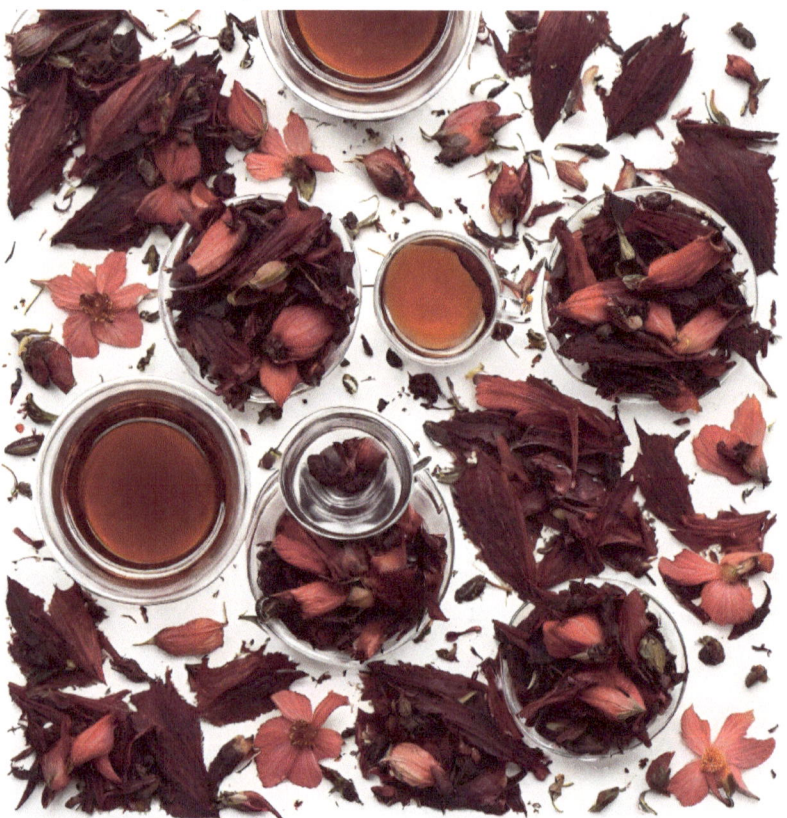

Ingredients:
1 hibiscus tea bag
1 rosehip tea bag
1 cup hot water
1 teaspoon honey (optional)

Directions:
- Steep hibiscus and rosehip tea bags in hot water for 5-7 minutes.
- Remove tea bags and sweeten with honey if desired.
- Sip on this vibrant herbal tea to support kidney wellness.

2. Nettle Leaf Infusion:

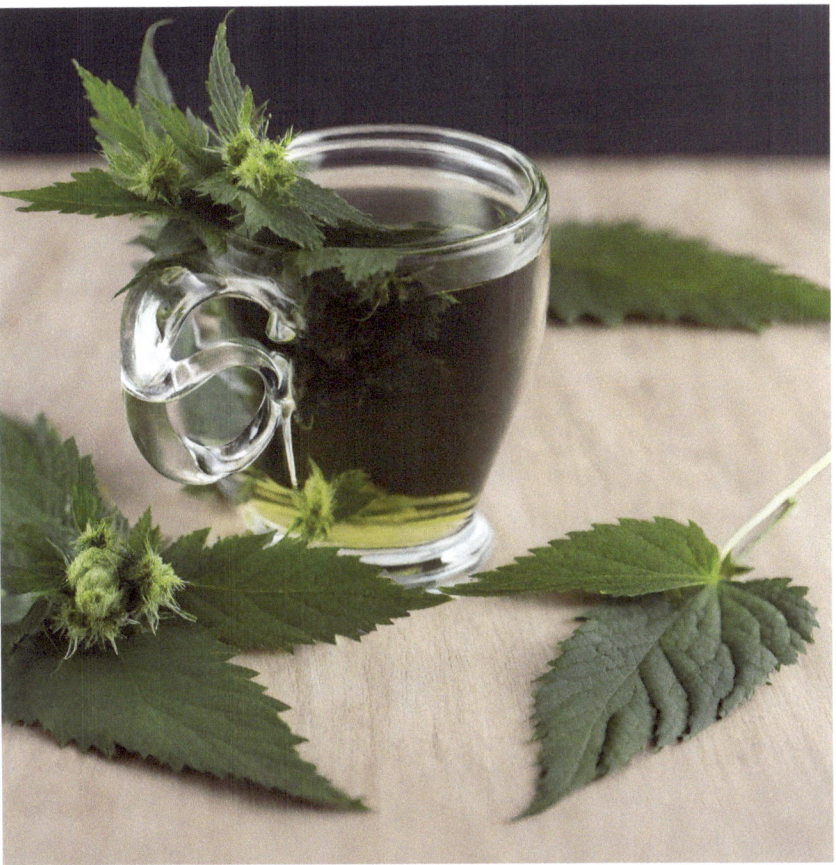

Ingredients:

1 tablespoon dried nettle leaves

1 cup hot water

1 slice lemon (optional)

Directions:

- Place dried nettle leaves in a cup.
- Pour hot water over the nettle leaves and let steep for 10 minutes.
- Strain, add a slice of lemon if desired, and enjoy this nourishing nettle leaf infusion.

These hydrating and kidney-supportive drinks are not only refreshing but also contribute to your overall well-being. Whether you opt for a citrus mint infusion, a berry blast smoothie, or a calming herbal tea, each sip is a step toward optimal hydration and renal health. Enjoy these beverages as part of your daily routine to stay refreshed and support your kidneys.

Chapter 8: Meal Plans and Weekly Menus

Sample Meal Plans for a Week

Embark on a week of balanced and kidney-friendly meals with these sample meal plans. Adjust portions based on individual needs, and remember to consult with a healthcare professional or nutritionist for personalized guidance.

Day 1

Breakfast - Oatmeal with Berries and Almonds:

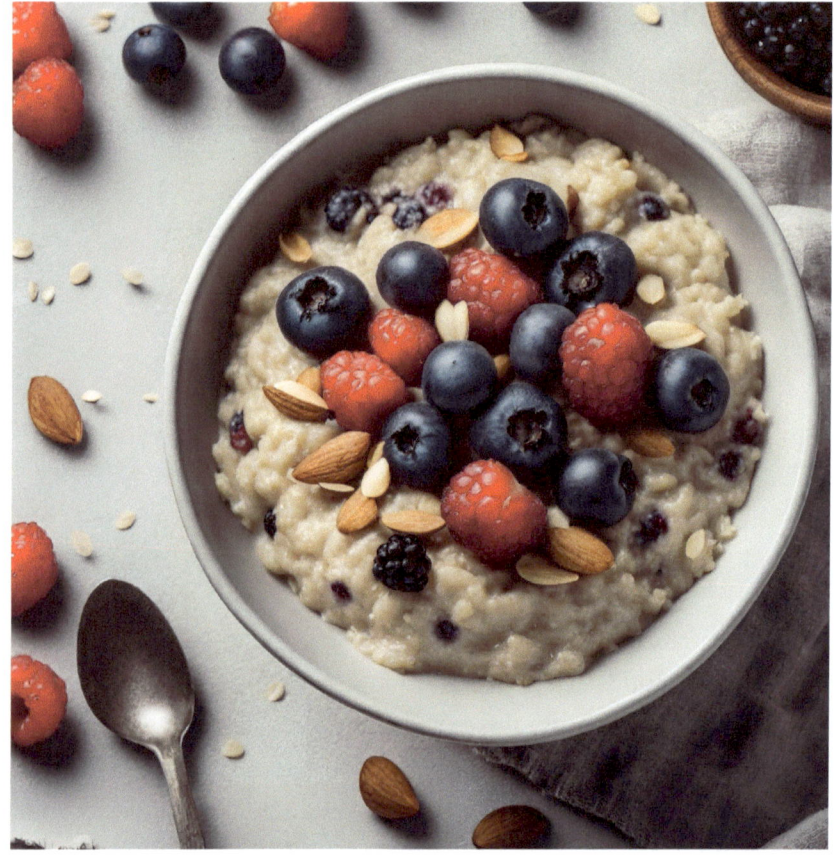

Serve: 1 bowl

Prep Time: 5 minutes

Cook Time: 10 minutes

Ingredients:

- 1/2 cup rolled oats
- 1 cup low-fat milk
- Mixed berries (strawberries, blueberries, raspberries)
- Sliced almonds

Directions:

1. Cook Oats:
    - In a saucepan, combine rolled oats and low-fat milk.
    - Cook over medium heat, stirring occasionally, until oats are creamy.
2. Prepare Toppings:
    - Wash and slice the berries.
    - Toast sliced almonds in a dry pan until golden.
3. Assemble:
    - Pour the cooked oats into a bowl.
    - Top with mixed berries and toasted almonds.

Lunch - Chicken and Vegetable Stir-Fry:

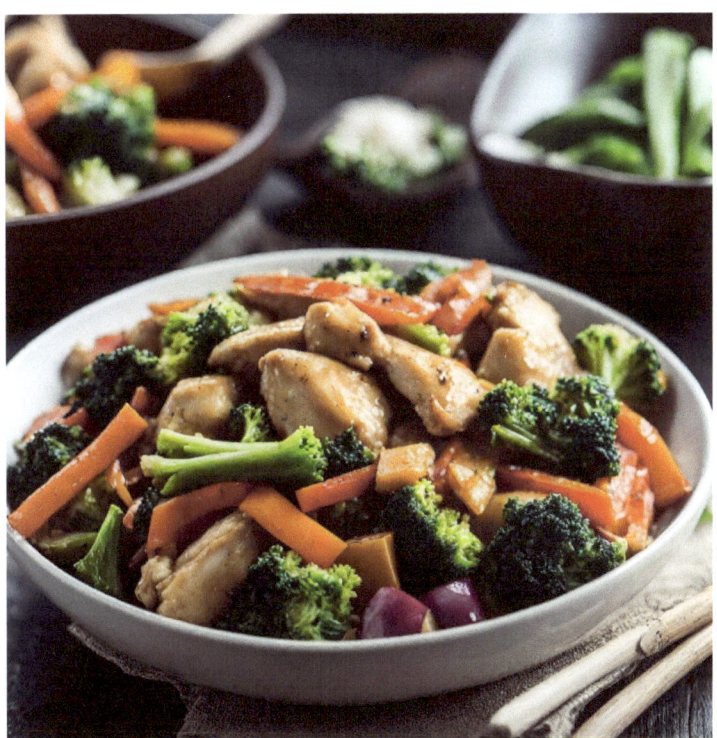

Serve: 1 plate

Prep Time: 15 minutes

Cook Time: 15 minutes

Ingredients:

- 4 oz chicken breast, sliced
- 1 cup broccoli florets
- 1 bell pepper, sliced
- 2 tbsp low-sodium soy sauce
- Olive oil

Directions:

1. Prepare Chicken:
   - Heat olive oil in a pan.
   - Cook sliced chicken until browned.
2. Add Vegetables:
   - Add broccoli and bell pepper to the pan.
   - Stir-fry until vegetables are tender.
3. Season:
   - Pour low-sodium soy sauce over the mixture.
   - Stir well to coat evenly.
4. Serve:
   - Transfer the stir-fry to a plate and serve.

Dinner - Baked Salmon with Quinoa and Asparagus:

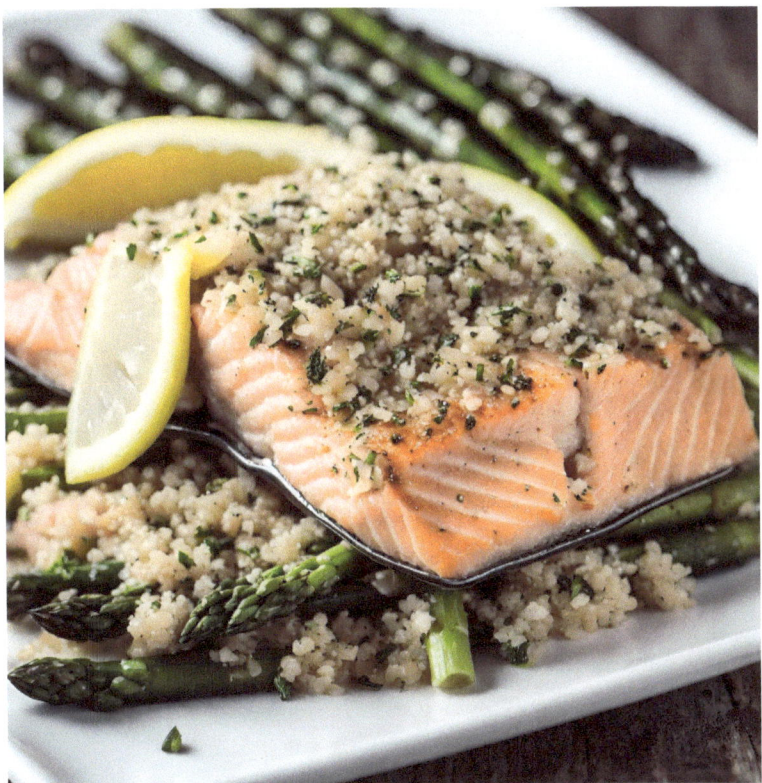

Serve: 1 serving

Prep Time: 10 minutes

Cook Time: 20 minutes

Ingredients:

- 1 salmon filet (about 6 oz)
- 1/2 cup quinoa
- 8-10 asparagus spears
- 1 lemon
- Fresh herbs (such as dill or parsley)
- Olive oil
- Salt and pepper to taste

Directions:

1. Preheat the Oven:

- Preheat your oven to 375°F (190°C).
2. Prepare the Salmon:
   - Rinse the salmon fillet under cold water and pat it dry with paper towels.
   - Place the salmon on a baking sheet lined with parchment paper.
3. Season the Salmon:
   - Drizzle olive oil over the salmon to prevent sticking.
   - Squeeze half of the lemon over the salmon.
   - Season with salt, pepper, and fresh herbs of your choice.
4. Prepare the Quinoa:
   - Rinse the quinoa under cold water.
   - In a saucepan, combine 1 cup of water and the rinsed quinoa. Bring to a boil.
   - Reduce heat, cover, and simmer for about 15 minutes or until the quinoa is cooked and water is absorbed.
5. Prepare the Asparagus:
   - Trim the woody ends of the asparagus.
   - Place asparagus on the baking sheet next to the salmon.
   - Drizzle with olive oil, sprinkle with salt and pepper.
6. Bake:
   - Place the baking sheet in the preheated oven.
   - Bake for 15-20 minutes or until the salmon easily flakes with a fork and the asparagus is tender.
7. Plate the Meal:
   - Fluff the cooked quinoa with a fork and place it on the plate.
   - Top with the baked salmon and arrange the roasted asparagus on the side.
   - Squeeze the remaining lemon over the dish for added freshness.
8. Garnish and Serve:
   - Garnish the dish with additional fresh herbs.
   - Serve immediately and enjoy your kidney-friendly, balanced meal!

Note: Ensure that the salmon reaches a minimum internal temperature of 145°F (63°C) for safe consumption. Adjust seasoning and ingredients based on personal preferences and dietary restrictions.

Day 2

Breakfast - Spinach and Feta Omelette:

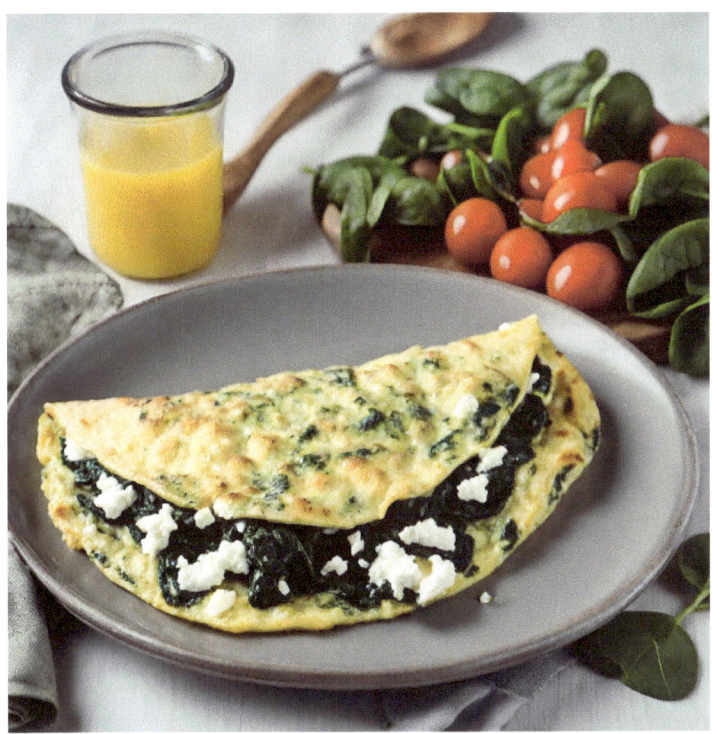

Serve: 1 Omelet

Prep Time: 10 minutes

Cook Time: 5 minutes

Ingredients:

- 2 eggs
- Handful of fresh spinach
- 1/4 cup crumbled feta cheese
- Olive oil

Directions:

1. Whisk Eggs:
   - In a bowl, whisk eggs until well combined.
2. Cook Spinach:
   - Heat olive oil in a pan.

- Add fresh spinach and sauté until wilted.

3. Add Eggs:
   - Pour whisked eggs over the spinach.
   - Allow eggs to set slightly.
4. Add Feta:
   - Sprinkle crumbled feta cheese over one half of the omelette.
5. Fold and Serve:
   - Fold the omelet in half.
   - Slide onto a plate and serve.

Lunch - Lentil Soup with Vegetables:

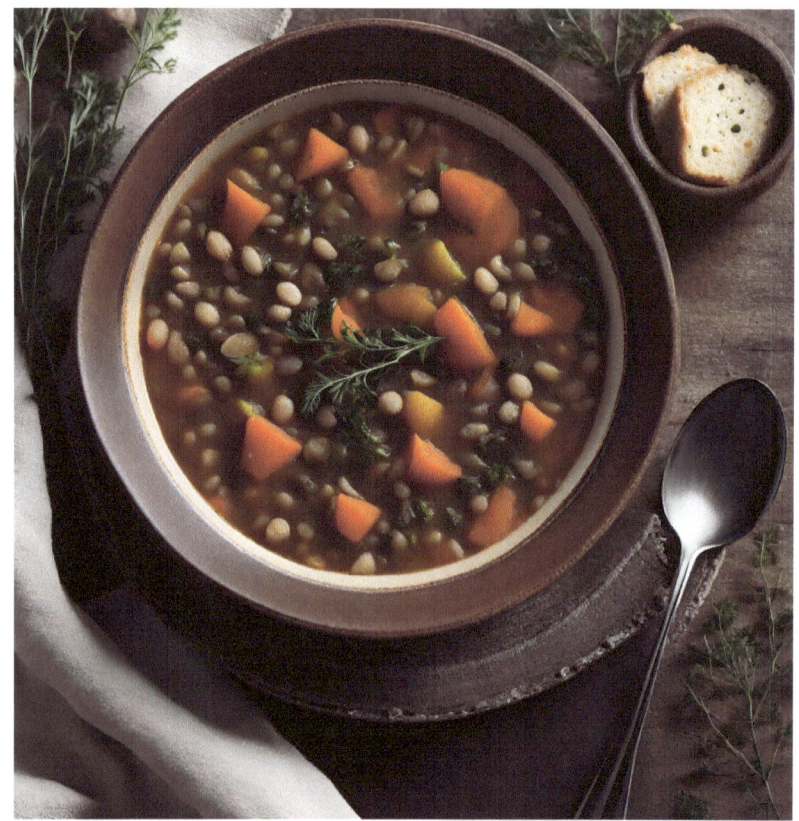

Serve: 1 bowl

Prep Time: 15 minutes

Cook Time: 30 minutes

Ingredients:

- 1/2 cup dried lentils
- 1 carrot, diced
- 1 celery stalk, diced
- 1/2 onion, chopped
- 2 cups low-sodium vegetable broth
- Garlic, minced
- Herbs (thyme, bay leaves)

Directions:

1. Sauté Vegetables:
   - In a pot, sauté chopped onion, diced carrot, and celery until softened.
2. Add Lentils:
   - Rinse lentils and add them to the pot.
   - Stir well.
3. Pour Broth:
   - Pour in low-sodium vegetable broth.
   - Add minced garlic and herbs.
4. Simmer:
   - Bring to a boil, then reduce heat and simmer until lentils are tender.
5. Season:
   - Season with salt and pepper to taste.
   - Remove bay leaves before serving.

Dinner - Grilled Chicken with Sweet Potato Mash:

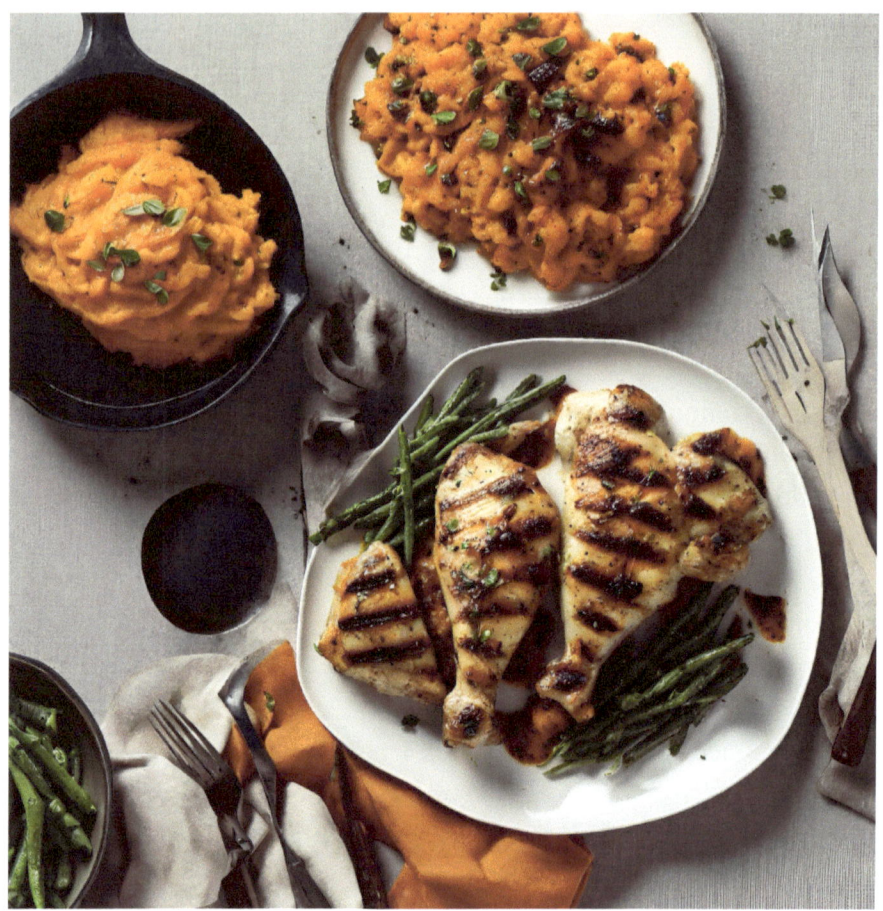

Serve: 1 plate

Prep Time: 20 minutes

Cook Time: 25 minutes

Ingredients:

- 6 oz chicken thighs
- 2 medium sweet potatoes
- Olive oil
- Garlic, minced
- Salt and pepper to taste

Directions:

1. Marinate Chicken:
   - Season chicken thighs with salt, pepper, and minced garlic.
   - Let it marinate for 10 minutes.
2. Grill Chicken:

   Grill chicken thighs until fully cooked, about 12-15 minutes.

3. Prepare Sweet Potato Mash:
   - Peel and chop sweet potatoes. Boil until tender.
   - Mash with a fork and season with salt and pepper.
4. Serve:
   - Plate the grilled chicken alongside the sweet potato mash.
   - Drizzle with olive oil and serve.

Note: Adjust portion sizes based on individual dietary needs. Consult a healthcare professional for personalized advice on kidney-friendly meals

Day 3

Breakfast - Greek Yogurt Parfait:

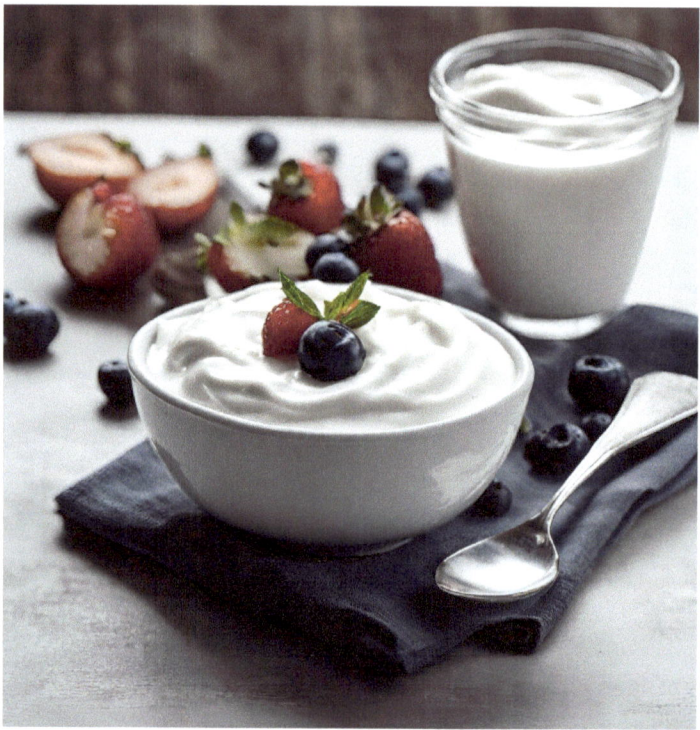

Serve: 1 bowl

Prep Time: 5 minutes

Cook Time: 0 minutes

Ingredients:

- Greek yogurt
- Fresh berries (strawberries, blueberries, raspberries)
- Honey
- Granola

Directions:

1. Layer Yogurt:
   - In a bowl or glass, start by adding a layer of Greek yogurt.
2. Add Berries:
   - Top the yogurt with a variety of fresh berries.

3. Drizzle with Honey:
   - Drizzle honey over the berries for sweetness.
4. Sprinkle Granola:
   - Finish by sprinkling granola on top for added crunch.
5. Serve:
   - Grab a spoon and enjoy your delightful and protein-packed Greek yogurt parfait.

Lunch - Quinoa and Black Bean Salad:

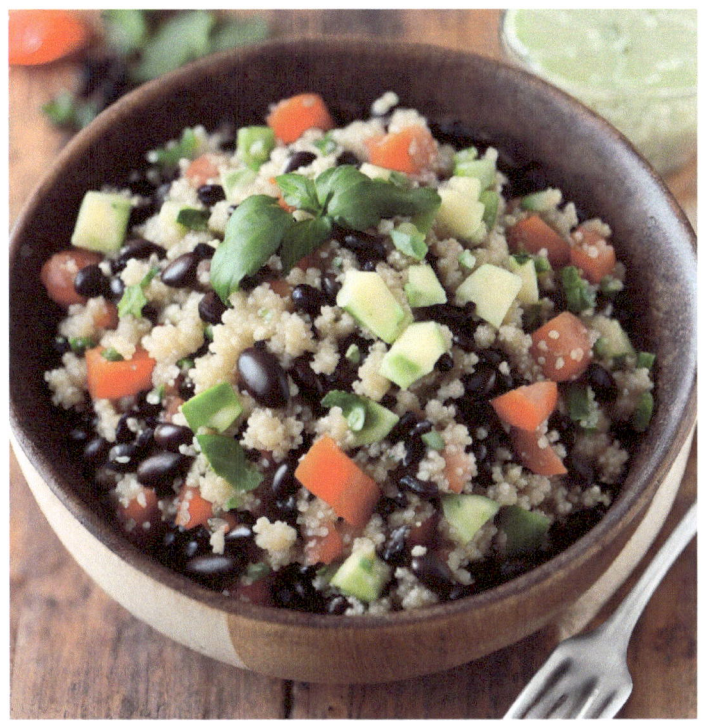

Serve: 1 plate

Prep Time: 20 minutes

Cook Time: 15 minutes

Ingredients:

- 1/2 cup quinoa
- 1/2 cup black beans (canned and drained)
- Corn kernels (fresh or canned)
- Bell peppers (assorted colors), diced
- Lime vinaigrette (lime juice, olive oil, salt, and pepper)

Directions:

1. Cook Quinoa:
   - Rinse quinoa under cold water.
   - In a saucepan, combine 1 cup of water and quinoa.
   - Bring to a boil, then simmer until water is absorbed.
2. Prepare Vegetables:
   - Dice bell peppers and gather corn kernels.
3. Mix Ingredients:
   - In a large bowl, combine cooked quinoa, black beans, bell peppers, and corn.
4. Make Lime Vinaigrette:
   - In a small bowl, whisk together lime juice, olive oil, salt, and pepper.
5. Toss and Serve:
   - Pour the lime vinaigrette over the quinoa mixture.
   - Toss everything together. Serve chilled.

Dinner - Turkey and Vegetable Skewers with Brown Rice:

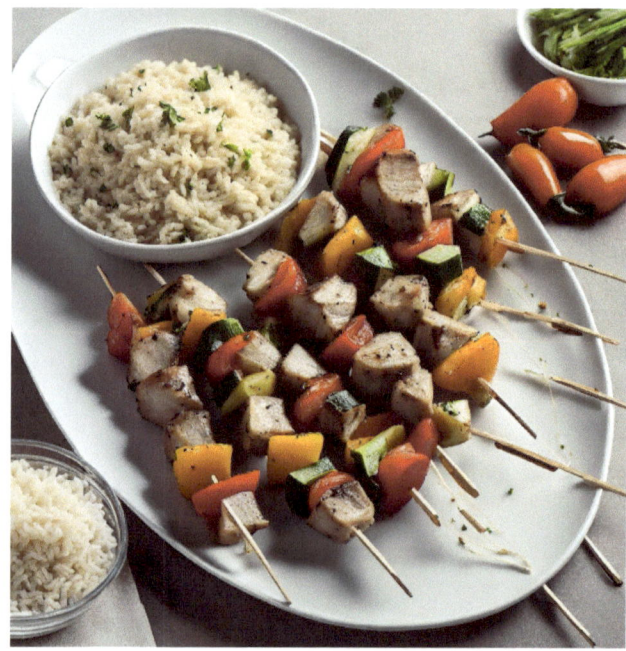

Serve: 1 plate

Prep Time: 25 minutes

Cook Time: 15 minutes

Ingredients:

- Turkey breast, cut into cubes
- Cherry tomatoes
- Zucchini, sliced
- Bell peppers (assorted colors), cut into chunks
- Olive oil
- Garlic powder, paprika, salt, and pepper
- Brown rice

Directions:

1. Prepare Skewers:
   - Thread turkey cubes, cherry tomatoes, zucchini slices, and bell pepper chunks onto skewers.
2. Season Skewers:
   - Drizzle olive oil over the skewers.
   - Sprinkle with garlic powder, paprika, salt, and pepper.
3. Grill or Broil:
   - Grill the skewers on an outdoor grill or broil in the oven until turkey is cooked and vegetables are slightly charred.
4. Cook Brown Rice:
   - While the skewers are cooking, prepare brown rice according to package instructions.
5. Serve:
   - Plate the cooked brown rice and top with turkey and vegetable skewers.
   - Enjoy this flavorful and nutritious dinner.

Note: Adjust portion sizes based on individual dietary needs. Consult a healthcare professional for personalized advice on kidney-friendly meals.

Day 4

Breakfast - Veggie Omelette with Whole Grain Toast

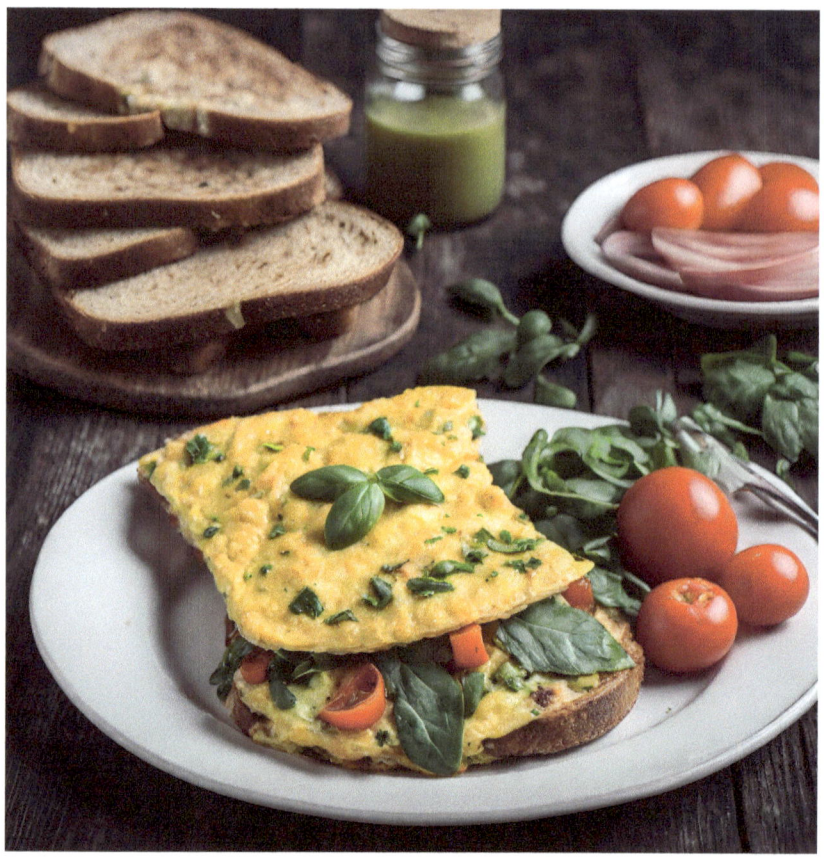

Serve: 1 Omelet , 1-2 slices of whole-grain toast

Prep Time: 15 minutes

Cook Time: 10 minutes

Ingredients:

- 2 eggs
- Bell peppers (assorted colors), diced
- Tomato, diced
- Onion, finely chopped
- Spinach, chopped
- Feta cheese (optional)
- Olive oil

- Salt and pepper to taste

Directions:

1. Whisk Eggs:
   - In a bowl, whisk the eggs until well beaten.
2. Sauté Vegetables:
   - Heat olive oil in a pan. Sauté diced bell peppers, tomatoes, and onions until softened.
   - Add chopped spinach and cook until wilted.
3. Pour Eggs:
   - Pour the whisked eggs over the sautéed vegetables in the pan.
4. Add Cheese (Optional):
   - Sprinkle feta cheese on one half of the omelette if desired.
5. Fold and Serve:
   - Once the eggs are set but still slightly runny on top, fold the omelette in half.
   - Cook until eggs are fully set. Serve with whole-grain toast.

Lunch - Chickpea Salad with Cucumber and Avocado:

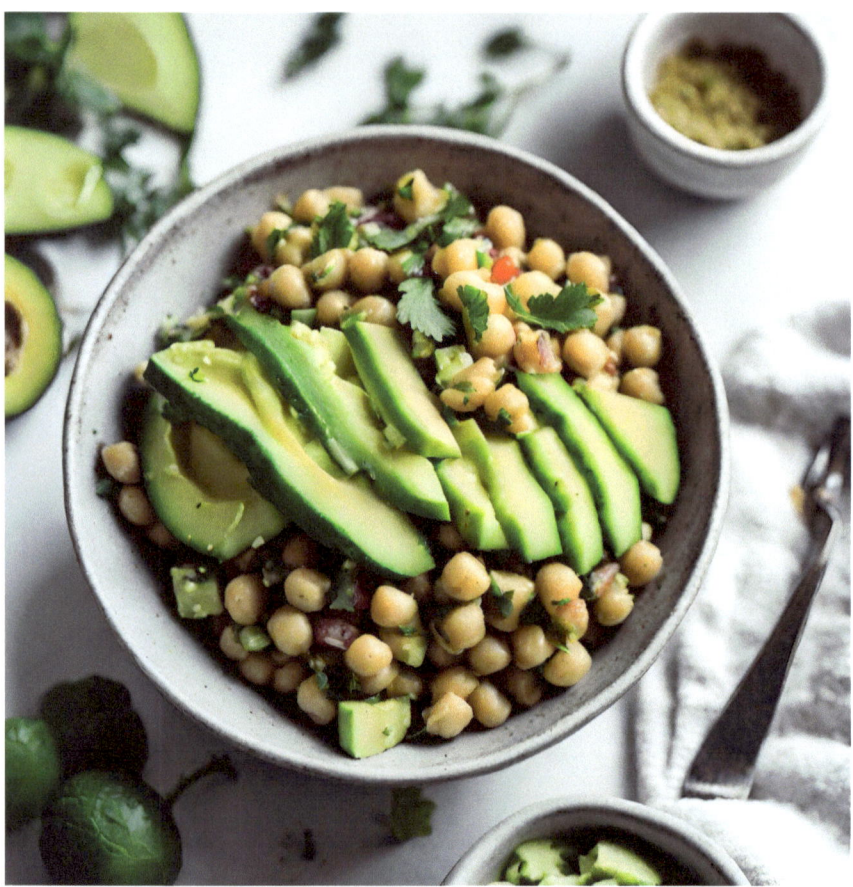

Serve: 1 bowl

Prep Time: 15 minutes

Cook Time: 0 minutes

Ingredients:

- 1 can chickpeas, drained and rinsed
- Cucumber, diced
- Avocado, diced
- Cherry tomatoes, halved
- Red onion, finely chopped
- Fresh cilantro, chopped
- Olive oil and lemon dressing

- Salt and pepper to taste

Directions:

1. Prepare Chickpeas:
   - Rinse canned chickpeas under cold water.
2. Combine Ingredients:
   - In a bowl, combine chickpeas, diced cucumber, avocado, cherry tomatoes, red onion, and fresh cilantro.
3. Make Dressing:
   - In a small bowl, whisk together olive oil, lemon juice, salt, and pepper.
4. Toss and Serve:
   - Pour the dressing over the salad.
   - Toss everything together and serve immediately.

Dinner - Shrimp Stir-Fry with Broccoli and Brown Rice:

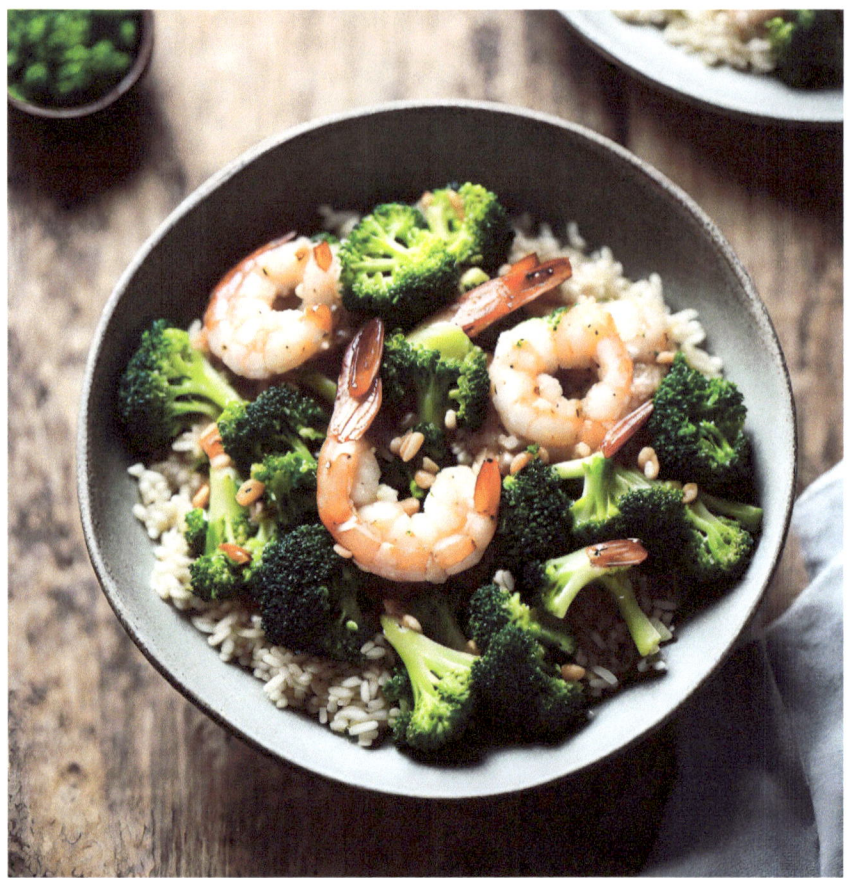

Serve: 1 plate

Prep Time: 20 minutes

Cook Time: 15 minutes

Ingredients:

- Shrimp, peeled and deveined
- Broccoli florets
- Carrots, sliced
- Snap peas
- Garlic, minced
- Soy sauce (low-sodium)
- Sesame oil
- Brown rice

Directions:

1. Cook Brown Rice:
   - Prepare brown rice according to package instructions.
2. Stir-Fry Shrimp:
   - In a wok or large pan, heat sesame oil.
   - Add shrimp and stir-fry until pink and cooked through.
   - Remove from the pan.
3. Sauté Vegetables:
   - In the same pan, add a bit more sesame oil.
   - Sauté broccoli, carrots, snap peas, and minced garlic until vegetables are tender-crisp.
4. Combine Ingredients:
   - Add the cooked shrimp back to the pan.
   - Pour in low-sodium soy sauce.
   - Stir-fry until everything is well combined.
5. Serve:
   - Plate the shrimp and vegetable stir-fry over cooked brown rice.
   - Enjoy this quick and flavorful dinner.

Note: Adjust portion sizes based on individual dietary needs. Consult a healthcare professional for personalized advice on kidney-friendly meals.

Day 5

Breakfast - Blueberry Banana Smoothie Bowl:

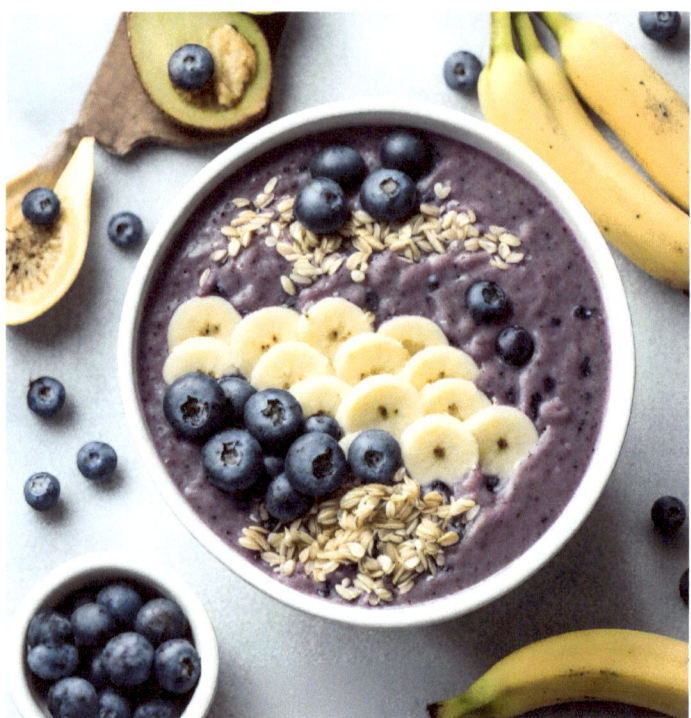

Serve: 1 bowl

Prep Time: 10 minutes

Cook Time: 0 minutes

Ingredients:

- 1 frozen banana
- 1/2 cup blueberries
- Greek yogurt
- Almond milk
- Chia seeds
- Granola

Directions:

1. Blend Smoothie Base:

In a blender, combine the frozen banana, blueberries, a dollop of Greek yogurt, and enough almond milk to achieve a thick smoothie consistency.

2. Pour into Bowl:
   - Pour the smoothie into a bowl.
3. Top with Goodies:
   - Sprinkle chia seeds and granola over the smoothie bowl.
4. Enjoy:
   - Grab a spoon and enjoy this refreshing and nutrient-packed breakfast.

Lunch - Spinach and Lentil Salad with Balsamic Vinaigrette:

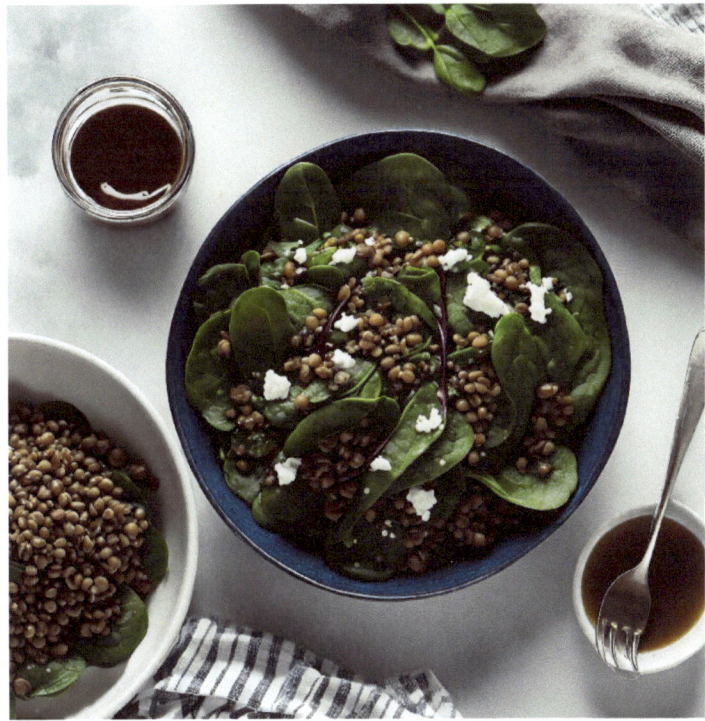

Serve: 1 bowl

Prep Time: 20 minutes

Cook Time: 20 minutes

Ingredients:

- 1/2 cup lentils, cooked
- Fresh spinach leaves
- Cherry tomatoes, halved

- Cucumber, sliced
- Red onion, thinly sliced
- Feta cheese, crumbled (optional)
- Balsamic vinaigrette

Directions:

1. Cook Lentils:
   - Cook lentils according to package instructions.
   - Allow them to cool.
2. Prepare Salad Base:
   - In a bowl, combine fresh spinach leaves, halved cherry tomatoes, sliced cucumber, and thinly sliced red onion.
3. Add Lentils:
   - Mix in the cooked and cooled lentils.
4. Top with Feta (Optional):
   - Sprinkle crumbled feta cheese over the salad.
5. Drizzle Dressing:
   - Pour balsamic vinaigrette over the salad and toss to combine.

Dinner - Grilled Vegetable and Chicken Skewers with Quinoa:

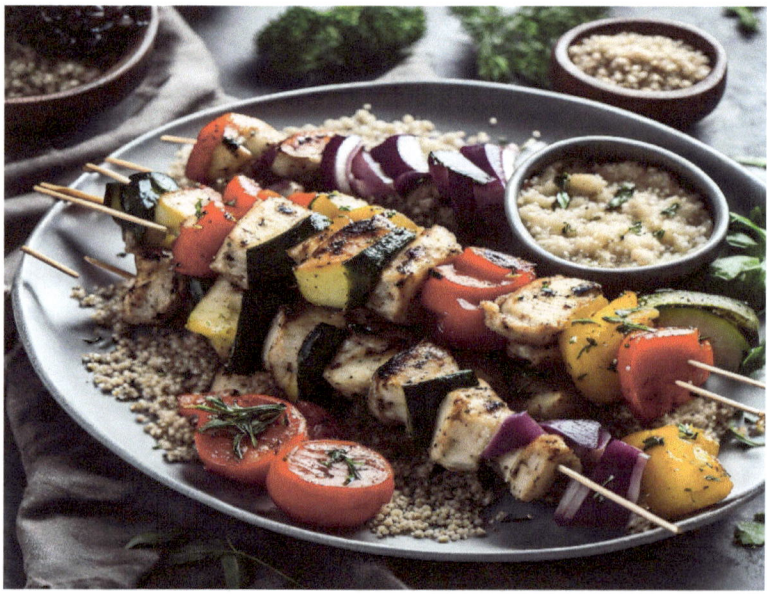

Serve: 1 plate

Prep Time: 30 minutes

Cook Time: 15 minutes

Ingredients:

- Chicken breast, cut into cubes
- Zucchini, sliced
- Cherry tomatoes
- Bell peppers (assorted colors), cut into chunks
- Red onion, cut into wedges
- Olive oil
- Garlic powder, dried oregano, salt, and pepper
- Quinoa, cooked

Directions:

1. Marinate Chicken:
   - In a bowl, combine chicken cubes with olive oil, garlic powder, dried oregano, salt, and pepper.
   - Let it marinate for at least 15 minutes.
2. Prepare Vegetables:
   - Thread marinated chicken, zucchini slices, cherry tomatoes, bell pepper chunks, and red onion wedges onto skewers.
3. Grill or Broil:
   - Grill the skewers on an outdoor grill or broil in the oven until chicken is fully cooked and vegetables are slightly charred.
4. Cook Quinoa:
   - While the skewers are cooking, prepare quinoa according to package instructions.
5. Serve:
   - Plate the cooked quinoa and top with grilled vegetable and chicken skewers.
   - Drizzle with a little olive oil if desired. Enjoy this colorful and wholesome dinner.

Note: Adjust portion sizes based on individual dietary needs. Consult a healthcare professional for personalized advice on kidney-friendly meals.

Day 6:

Breakfast - Chia Seed Pudding with Fresh Fruit:

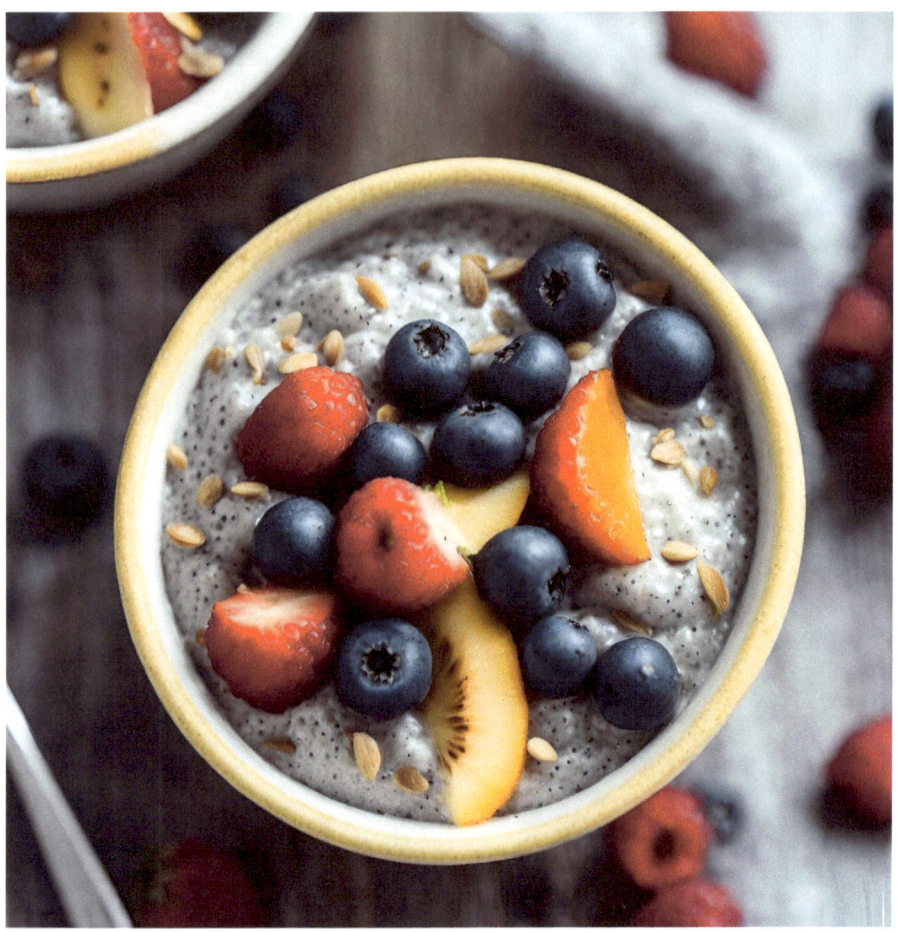

Serve: 1 bowl

Prep Time: 5 minutes (plus overnight soaking)

Cook Time: 0 minutes

Ingredients:

- 2 tablespoons chia seeds
- 1/2 cup almond milk
- Fresh berries (strawberries, raspberries, blueberries)
- Sliced banana
- Drizzle of honey

Directions:

1. Mix Chia Seeds and Milk:
   - In a bowl, combine chia seeds and almond milk.
   - Stir well and refrigerate overnight or for at least 4 hours until it forms a pudding-like consistency.
2. Layer with Fresh Fruit:
   - Once the chia seed pudding is set, layer it with fresh berries and sliced banana.
3. Drizzle with Honey:
   - Finish by drizzling honey over the top for sweetness.
4. Enjoy:
   - Grab a spoon and savor this nutritious and filling breakfast.

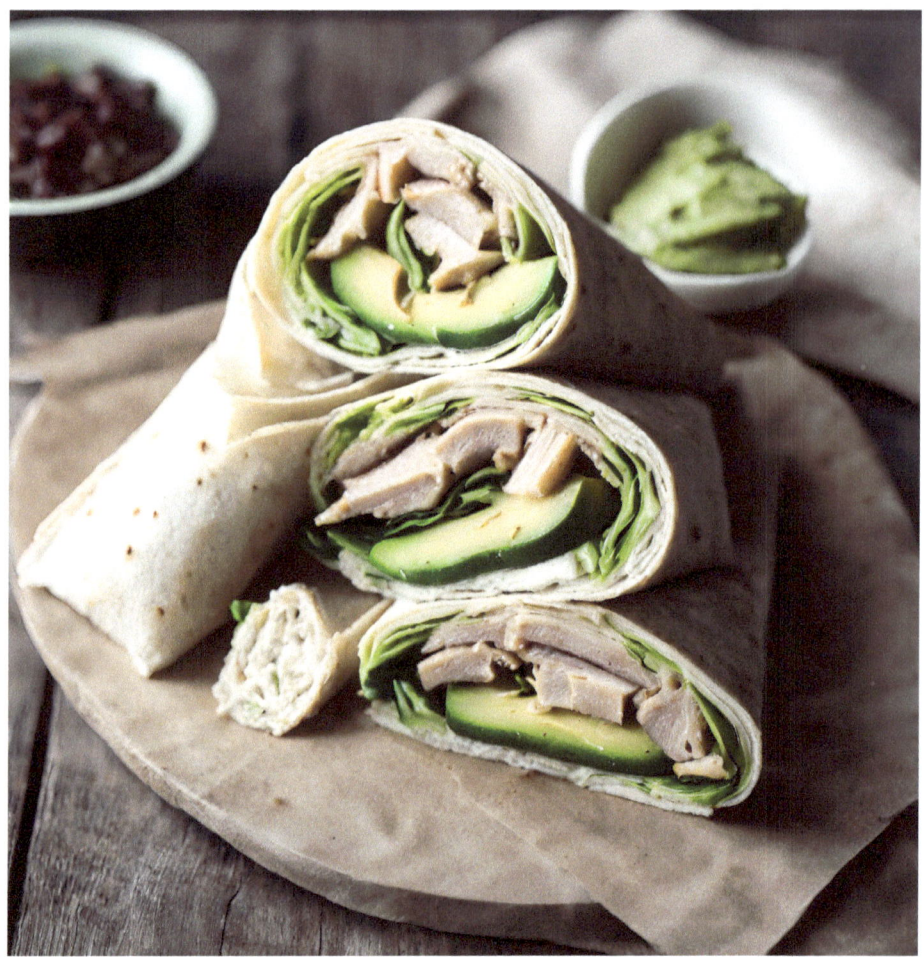

Serve: 1 wrap

Prep Time: 15 minutes

Cook Time: 0 minutes

Ingredients:

- Whole-grain wrap
- Sliced turkey breast
- Avocado, sliced
- Cherry tomatoes, halved
- Lettuce leaves
- Greek yogurt or light mayo
- Mustard

- Salt and pepper to taste

Directions:

1. Prepare Wrap Base:
   - Lay out the whole-grain wrap on a clean surface.
2. Layer Ingredients:
   - Place sliced turkey breast, avocado slices, cherry tomatoes, and lettuce leaves in the center of the wrap.
3. Add Sauces:
   - Spread a thin layer of Greek yogurt or light mayo and a dash of mustard over the ingredients.
4. Season and Wrap:
   - Season with salt and pepper to taste.
   - Wrap the ingredients tightly into a burrito-style wrap.
5. Serve:
   - Slice the wrap in half if desired and serve.

Dinner - Baked Cod with Lemon and Herbs, Quinoa, and Steamed Broccoli:

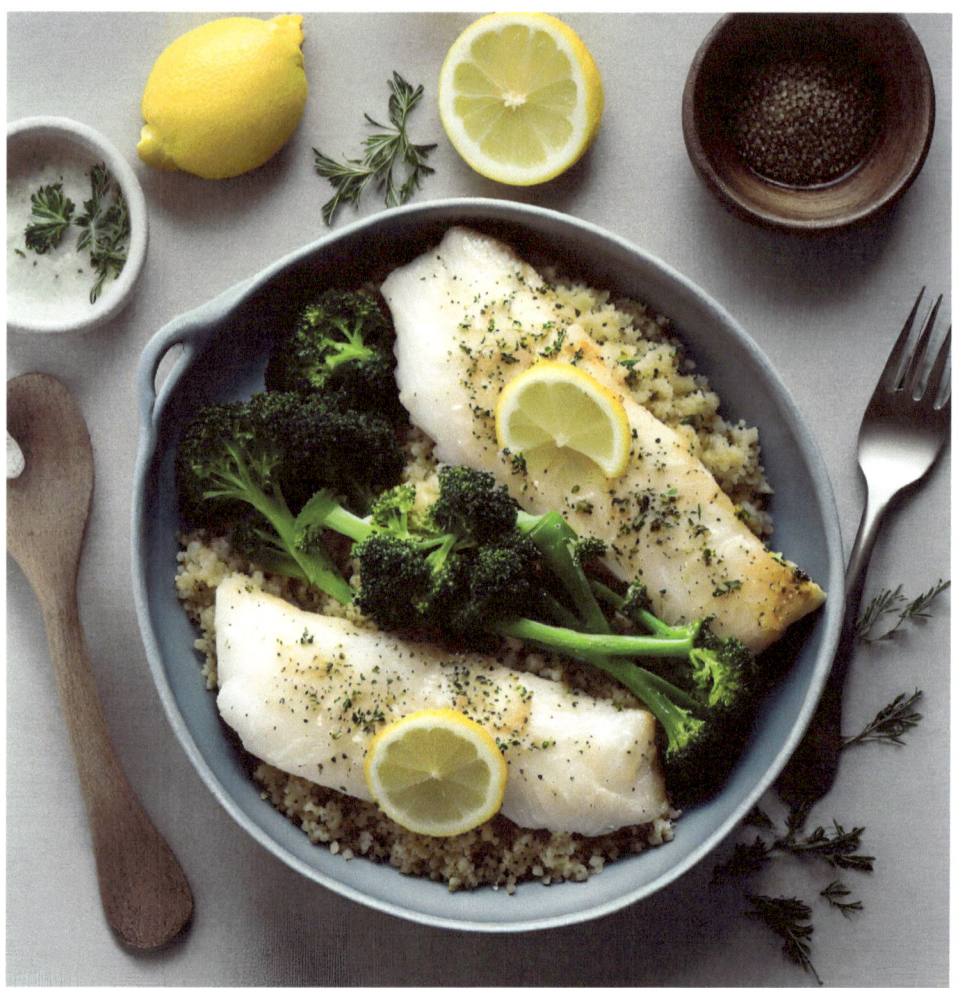

Serve: 1 plate

Prep Time: 15 minutes

Cook Time: 20 minutes

Ingredients:

- Cod fillet
- Lemon
- Fresh herbs (parsley, dill)
- Olive oil
- Quinoa, cooked
- Broccoli florets

Directions:

1. Preheat the Oven:
   - Preheat your oven to 375°F (190°C).
2. Prepare Cod:
   - Place the cod fillet on a baking sheet lined with parchment paper.
   - Drizzle olive oil over the cod.
   - Squeeze lemon juice over the fish and sprinkle with fresh herbs.
3. Bake Cod:
   - Bake in the preheated oven for about 15-20 minutes or until the fish flakes easily with a fork.
4. Prepare Quinoa:
   - While the cod is baking, reheat or cook quinoa according to package instructions.
5. Steam Broccoli:
   - Steam broccoli florets until they are tender-crisp.
6. Serve:
   - Plate the baked cod over a bed of quinoa.
   - Arrange steamed broccoli on the side.
   - Drizzle a bit of lemon juice over the entire dish and garnish with additional fresh herbs if desired.

Note: Adjust portion sizes based on individual dietary needs. Consult a healthcare professional for personalized advice on kidney-friendly meals.

Day 7

Breakfast - Overnight Oats with Nut Butter and Banana:

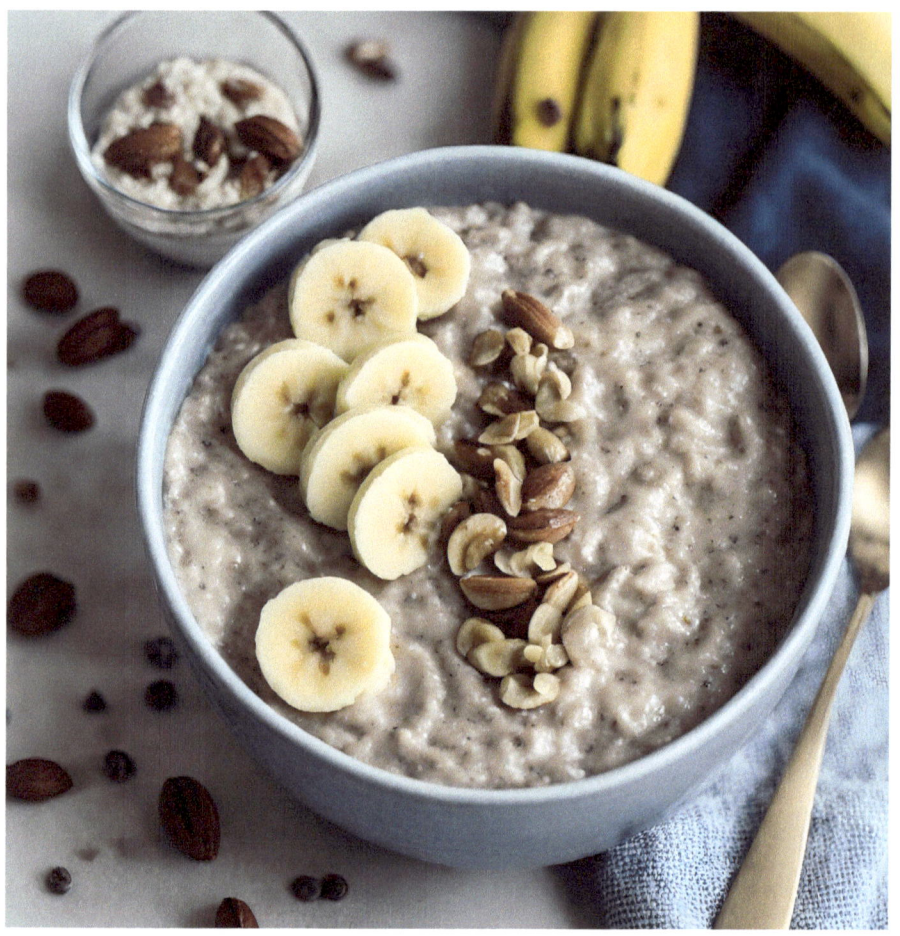

Serve: 1 bowl

Prep Time: 5 minutes (plus overnight soaking)

Cook Time: 0 minutes

Ingredients:

- 1/2 cup rolled oats
- 1/2 cup almond milk
- 1 tablespoon nut butter (almond, peanut, or your choice)
- Sliced banana
- Chopped nuts (walnuts, almonds)
- Drizzle of honey

Directions:

1. Combine Oats and Milk:
   - In a jar or bowl, mix rolled oats and almond milk.
   - Stir well and refrigerate overnight or for at least 4 hours until oats absorb the liquid.
2. Layer with Nut Butter and Banana:
   - Once the oats are ready, layer the top with nut butter, sliced banana, and chopped nuts.
3. Drizzle with Honey:
   - Finish by drizzling honey over the top for added sweetness.
4. Stir and Enjoy:
   - Give it a good stir to combine all the flavors and enjoy this convenient and nutritious breakfast.

Lunch - Quinoa Stuffed Bell Peppers:

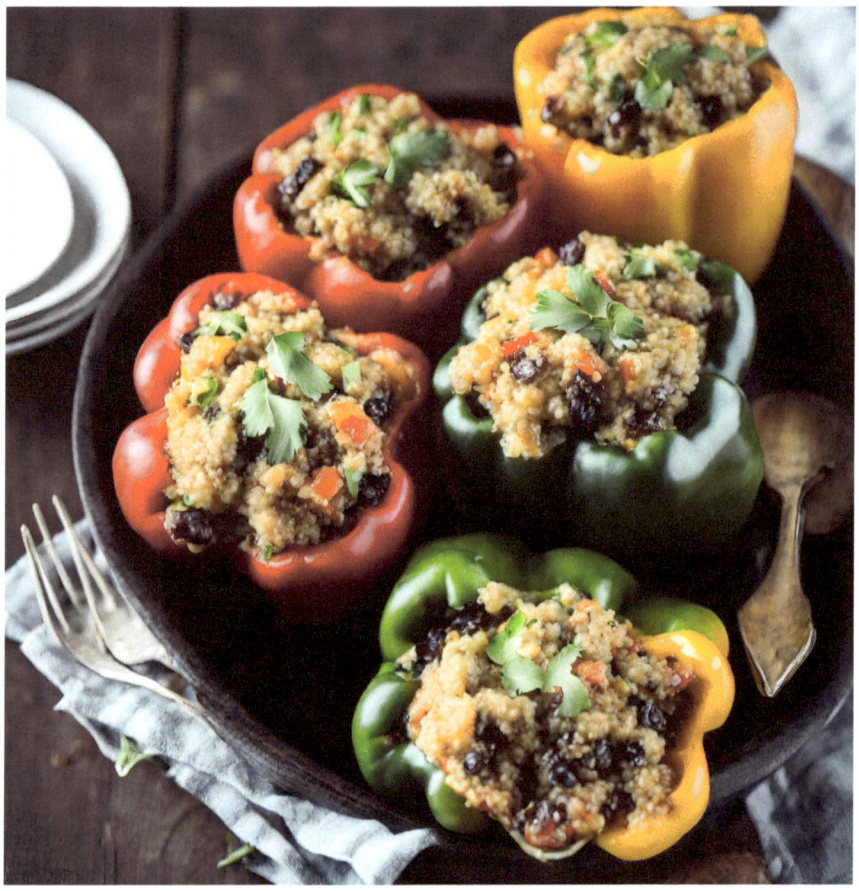

Serve: 2 stuffed bell peppers

Prep Time: 30 minutes

Cook Time: 25 minutes

Ingredients:

- 1 cup quinoa, cooked
- Lean ground turkey or chicken
- Bell peppers (assorted colors), halved
- Black beans, drained and rinsed
- Corn kernels
- Onion, diced
- Garlic, minced
- Tomato sauce
- Mexican seasoning (cumin, chili powder, paprika)

- Shredded cheese (cheddar or Mexican blend)

Directions:

1. Preheat the Oven:
   - Preheat your oven to 375°F (190°C).
2. Prepare Quinoa:
   - Cook quinoa according to package instructions.
3. Sauté Ground Turkey:
   - In a pan, cook lean ground turkey until browned. Add diced onion and minced garlic.
4. Combine Ingredients:
   - In a large bowl, mix cooked quinoa, sautéed ground turkey, black beans, corn, tomato sauce, and Mexican seasoning.
5. Prepare Bell Peppers:
   - Cut bell peppers in half and remove seeds and membranes.
   - Stuff each half with the quinoa and turkey mixture.
6. Bake:
   - Place the stuffed bell peppers in a baking dish.
   - Top each stuffed pepper with shredded cheese.
   - Bake Until Cheese Melts:
   - Bake in the preheated oven for about 25 minutes or until the cheese is melted and bubbly.
7. Serve:
   - Remove from the oven and serve the quinoa-stuffed bell peppers warm.

Dinner - Eggplant and Chickpea Curry with Brown Rice:

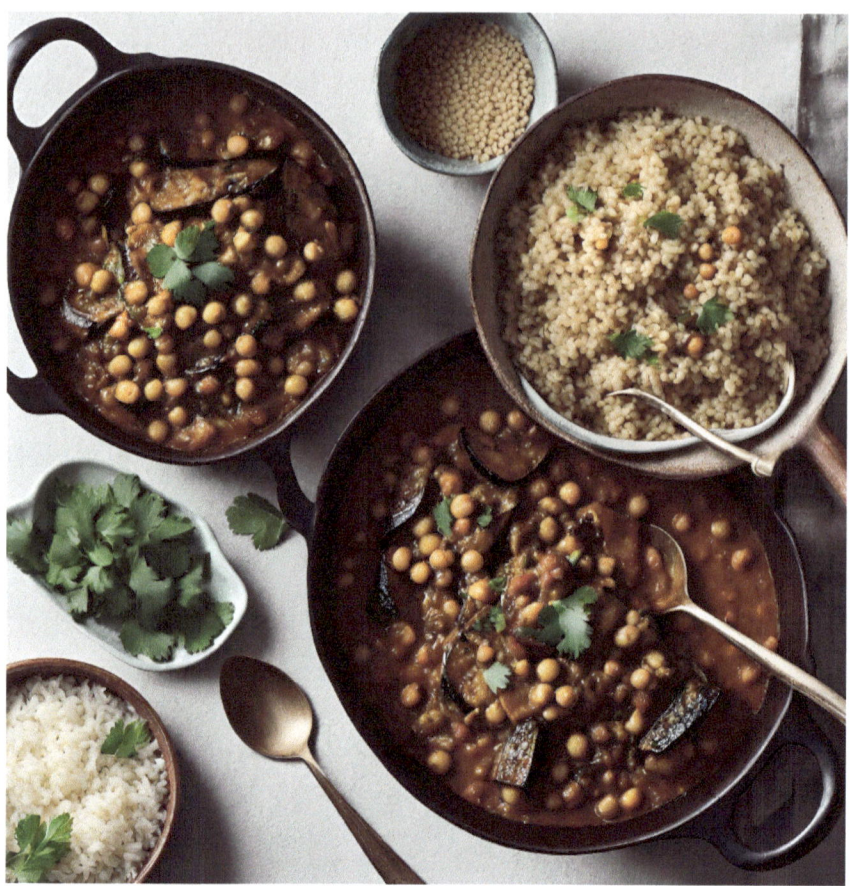

Serve: 1 plate

Prep Time: 20 minutes

Cook Time: 30 minutes

Ingredients:

- Eggplant, diced
- Chickpeas, cooked
- Onion, finely chopped
- Garlic, minced
- Ginger, grated
- Tomato, chopped
- Coconut milk
- Curry powder, cumin, coriander, turmeric
- Brown rice, cooked

Directions:

1. Sauté Aromatics:
   - In a pot, sauté finely chopped onion, minced garlic, and grated ginger until fragrant.
2. Add Vegetables:
   - Add diced eggplant and cook until softened.
3. Stir in Spices:
   - Stir in curry powder, cumin, coriander, and turmeric. Cook for a couple of minutes.
4. Add Chickpeas and Tomatoes:
   - Add cooked chickpeas and chopped tomatoes to the pot.
5. Pour Coconut Milk:
   - Pour in coconut milk. Simmer until the curry thickens.
6. Season and Serve:
   - Season with salt and pepper to taste.
   - Serve the eggplant and chickpea curry over cooked brown rice.
7. Garnish and Enjoy:
   - Garnish with fresh cilantro or parsley if desired.
   - Enjoy this flavorful and wholesome curry dish.

Note: Adjust portion sizes based on individual dietary needs. Consult a healthcare professional for personalized advice on kidney-friendly meals.

Chapter 9: Essential Kitchen Tips for Renal-Friendly Cooking

Using these vital kidney-friendly cooking guidelines, you can prioritize kidney health and cook with confidence in your kitchen.

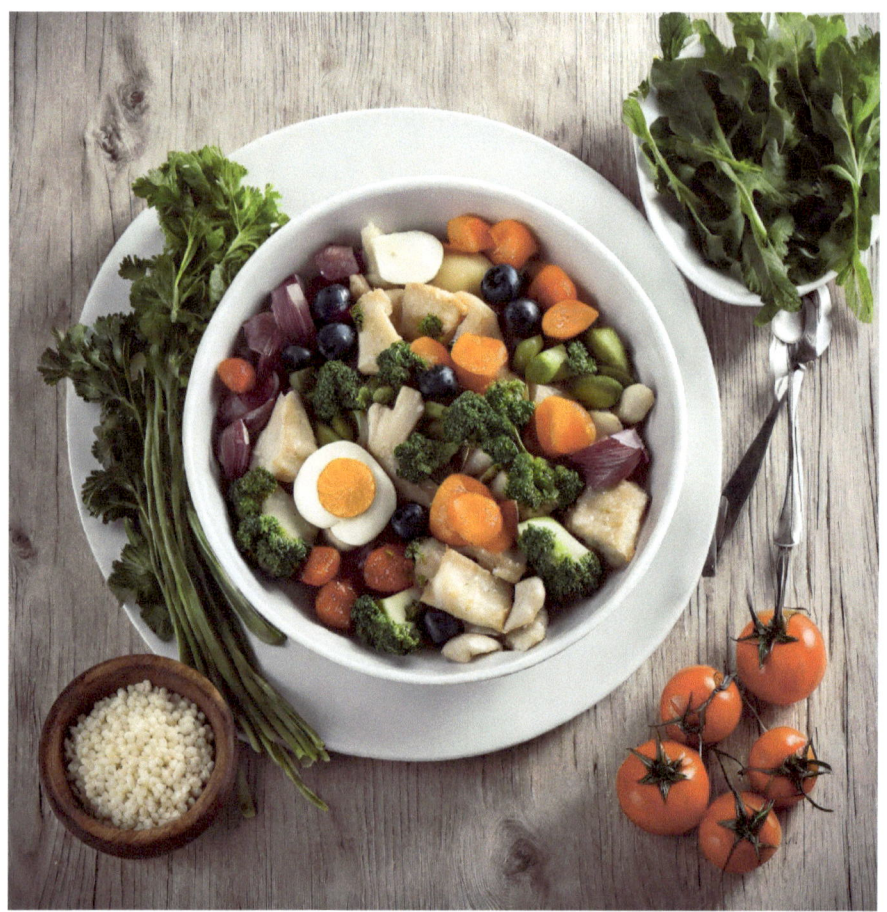

Methods for Reducing Sodium

Accept herbs and spices: Add flavor to your food with herbs like paprika and cumin, as well as spices like rosemary, thyme, and basil.

Zest and juice from citrus fruits: Add zest or juice from lemons, limes, or oranges to improve flavor without adding sodium.

Types of vinegar: To give your dishes more depth, try experimenting with different vinegars, such as apple cider or balsamic.

Low-sodium soups: To keep the sodium level in your meals under control, use homemade or low-sodium broths.

Purchasing Food Wisely to Maintain Kidney Health

Fresh produce: To guarantee a diet high in nutrients and suitable for renal function, give priority to a range of fresh fruits and vegetables.

Lean proteins: To promote kidney health, choose lean protein sources including fish, poultry, tofu, and lentils.

Whole grains: For more fiber and minerals, choose whole grains like brown rice, quinoa, and whole wheat pasta.

Options low in sodium: Opt for reduced-sodium or sodium-free varieties of sauces, condiments, and canned foods.

Examining labels: Check food labels carefully for any hidden sodium content and stay away from additives with high sodium concentration.

Meal Preparation and Portion Management

To satisfy your nutritional requirements, create balanced meals that feature a range of nutrient-dense foods.

Recognizing portions: Pay attention to portion sizes to prevent consuming too much of some nutrients, particularly protein and sodium.

Balanced plate: To guarantee a well-rounded diet, arrange a variety of lean proteins, nutritious grains, and vibrant veggies on your plates.

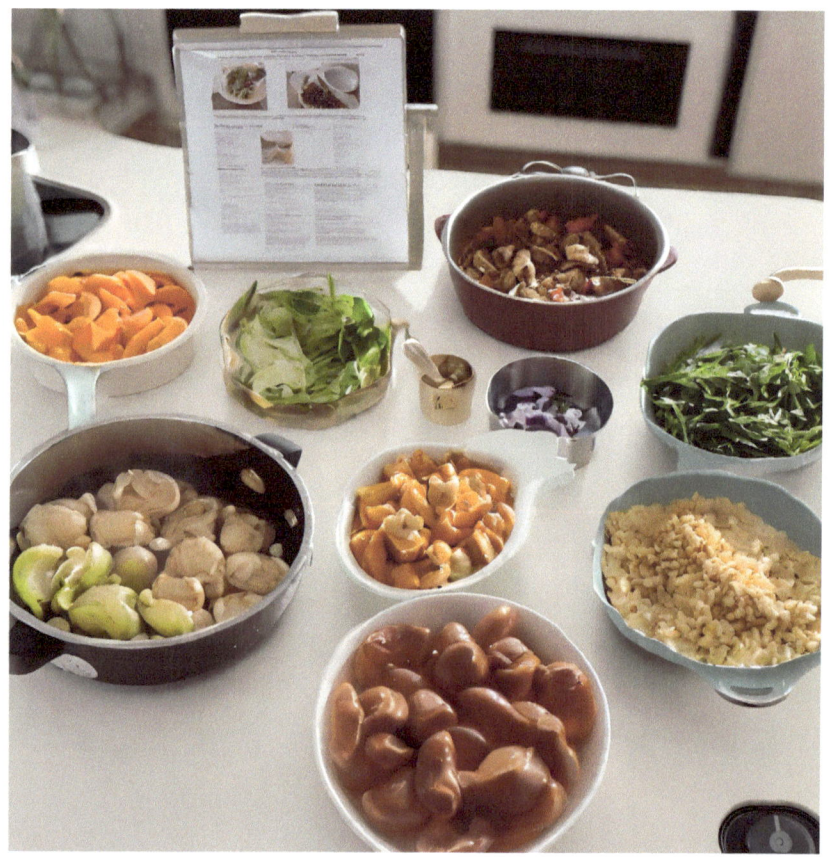

Cooking Methods for Kidney–Friendly Results

Steaming: Retain nutrients while minimizing added fats by incorporating steaming into your cooking routine.

Grilling without charring: Grill proteins and vegetables without charring to reduce the formation of harmful compounds.

Baking and roasting: Utilize baking and roasting for flavorful dishes with minimal added fats. Stir-frying with moderation: Employ stir-frying sparingly and use minimal oil to keep sodium levels in check.

By integrating these kitchen tips into your culinary practices, you embark on a journey of delicious and kidney-friendly cooking. These strategies not only enhance the flavor of your meals but also contribute to the overall well-being of your kidneys.

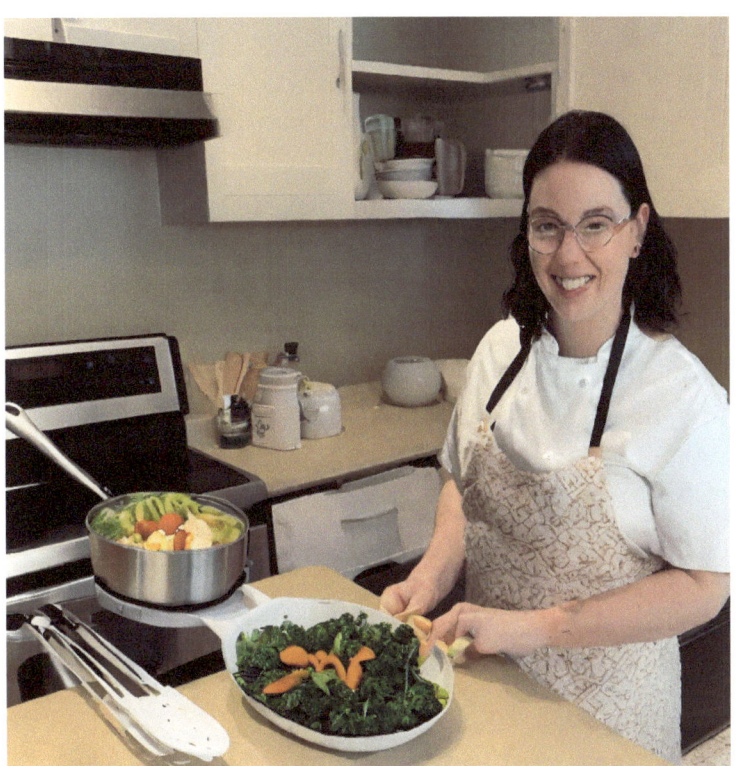

Conclusion

Celebrating Kidney-Friendly Cooking Success

Well done on your dedication to cooking kidney-friendly food! These observations on your gastronomic adventure and commitment to long-term renal health are a wonderful way to honor your accomplishments.

Delightful Accomplishments:
Appreciate the bright flavors you've added to your food without depending too much on salt.
Celebrate becoming an expert at enhancing the flavor of your food with herbs, spices, and other natural ingredients.

Rich in Nutrients Triumphs:
Acknowledge your nutrient-dense decisions by include a wide variety of vibrant fruits, veggies, lean meats, and entire grains.
Congratulations! You've prepared meals that improve kidney health and enhance your overall health.

Creative Culinary Arts:
Celebrate the culinary ingenuity you've unlocked by trying out new dishes and modifying them to adhere to kidney-friendly guidelines.

Celebrate the joy of discovering alternative ingredients and cooking techniques that align with your commitment to lifelong kidney health.

Commitment to Lifelong Kidney Health:

Reflect on the long-term impact of your dedication to kidney health, recognizing that your culinary choices contribute to a healthier future.
Appreciate the resilience and determination you've shown in maintaining a kidney-friendly lifestyle.

Building Sustainable Habits:

Pat yourself on the back for establishing sustainable habits that prioritize renal wellness without compromising the joy of cooking and eating.

Celebrate the transformation of kidney-friendly cooking from a choice to a fulfilling and enjoyable part of your daily routine.

Empowering Others:

Recognize the potential impact of your journey on inspiring others to embark on their own path to kidney health.

Share your successes and lessons learned, contributing to a supportive community of individuals committed to lifelong kidney well-being.

Remember, celebrating your kidney-friendly cooking success is not just about the meals you've prepared but also about the positive impact on your health and the lives of those around you. Your commitment to lifelong kidney health is a journey worth celebrating, and each flavorful, nutrient-rich dish is a testament to your dedication and resilience. Cheers to the delicious and kidney-friendly road ahead!

Appendix

Quick Reference Guide: Low Sodium Substitutes

This fast reference book can help you improve your low-sodium cooking by providing choices to lower your salt intake without sacrificing flavor or culinary delight.

Spices and Herbs: For a stronger taste, try substituting herbs like paprika, garlic powder, thyme, or basil for salt.

Juices and Zest of Citrus: Zest or juice from citrus fruits, such as oranges, lemons, or limes, can add color to food without adding sodium.

Types of Vinegar: To give your dishes more depth and acidity, try experimenting with balsamic, apple cider, or rice vinegar.

Low-sodium broths: Use homemade or low-sodium broths to add flavor to soups, stews, and sauces.

Blends of Spices Made at Home: For a personalized touch, create your own spice blends with herbs, spices, and no-salt seasonings.

Dried or Fresh Herbs: Garnish dishes with fresh herbs like parsley, cilantro, or dill or use dried herbs for added aroma and taste.

Seeds and Nuts: Enhance texture and flavor by incorporating seeds (sesame, chia) and unsalted nuts into salads, cereals, or baked goods.

Homemade Sauces: Prepare sauces from scratch using fresh ingredients, reducing the need for store-bought, high-sodium alternatives.

Fresh Produce: Prioritize a colorful array of fresh fruits and vegetables to elevate nutritional value and taste.

Lean Proteins: Opt for lean protein sources like chicken, turkey, fish, tofu, and legumes to maintain protein intake with less sodium.

Glossary of Terms

Renal Wellness: Focus on practices that support kidney health and function.

Sodium Intake: The amount of sodium consumed through food and beverages, a critical factor in kidney health.

Flavor Infusion: Incorporating herbs, spices, and other natural ingredients to enhance the taste of dishes without relying on excess salt.

Nutrient-Rich Choices: Selecting foods that are rich in essential nutrients, promoting overall well-being.

Culinary Adaptation: Adjusting recipes to align with dietary restrictions or preferences, such as reducing sodium content.

Herbaceous Aroma: The pleasant and fragrant scent produced by fresh or dried herbs in cooking.

Acidity Balance: Achieving equilibrium in flavors by incorporating acidic elements like vinegar or citrus.

Custom Spice Blend: A mixture of herbs, spices, and seasonings crafted to suit personal taste preferences without relying on pre-packaged mixes.

This quick reference guide empowers you to navigate low sodium cooking with ease, offering a variety of substitutes and a glossary of terms to enhance your culinary journey towards kidney-friendly and flavorful meals.